IT WON'T
HAPPEN TO ME

Also by Susan Newman

Never Say Yes to a Stranger
You <u>Can</u> Say No to a Drink or a Drug

IT WON'T HAPPEN TO ME

SUSAN NEWMAN

Photographs by
George Tiboni

A Perigee Book

Perigee Books
are published by
The Putnam Publishing Group
200 Madison Avenue
New York, NY 10016

Library of Congress Cataloging-in-Publication Data

Newman, Susan.
  It won't happen to me.

  Summary: Case histories of nine teenage alcoholics and drug
addicts, illustrating the problems of alcohol
and drug abuse among young people.
  1. Youth—United States—Alcohol use—Juvenile
literature.   2. Youth—United States—Drug use—
Juvenile literature.   3. Youth—United States—
Interviews—Juvenile literature.   [1. Drug abuse.
2. Alcoholism]   I. Tiboni, George, ill.   II. Title.
HV5066.N49   1987   362.2'92'088055   86-25503
ISBN 0-399-51342-6

Typeset by Fisher Composition, Inc.

Book design by The Sarabande Press

Printed in the United States of America

1   2   3   4   5   6   7   8   9   10

*To the special people who trusted me with the
very private and painful experiences of their
alcohol and drug dependency and whose openness
and honesty made this book possible.*

ACKNOWLEDGMENTS

Teens and parents alike need to understand the pitfalls of what is often passed off as innocent and harmless alcohol and drug use. For most, however, understanding comes during rehabilitation. Books and pamphlets that focus on dangers and problems suddenly become plentiful after the problems of abuse require professional help. Little exists that provides a clear picture of life in the alcohol/drug world *before* it's too late.

My sincere thanks go to those who helped fill this hazardous void:

—Sue Morrow of the Hunterdon Drug Awareness Program and Ruth Hague, an employee's assistance counselor, for making it possible for me to find the many young recovering and recovered alcoholics and drug addicts who were interviewed for this book.
—William Stender, executive director, Monmouth Chemical Dependency Treatment Center, for sharing his extensive knowledge.
—Thomas G. Matro, associate professor of English, Rutgers University, for astute observations and suggestions.
—Scott McGrath for his research assistance and sensitivity to the problems of convincing teenagers that drugs are dangerous.
—Those who contributed significantly to the photographic realism of the case histories: John F. Kennedy Hospital, Edison, N.J.; Metuchen Police Department; John R. Novak, principal, Metuchen High School; parents who let us into their homes; people who let us into their places of business; and

Nina McGrath, who kept the people and pieces together.

I am especially grateful to Judy Linden, my editor, for believing in and supporting this project completely, and to Alice Martell, my agent, for her warm professionalism.

CONTENTS

WHO ARE THE PEOPLE?   11

1. It Won't Happen to Me   15

2. Terry (First drink, age 14)   17

3. Kimberly (First drug, age 10)   27

4. Martin (First drink, age 13)   39

5. Sheila (First drink, age 9)   51

6. Courtney (First drug, age 14)   63

7. Gary (First drink, age 14)   74

8. Melissa (First drink, age 11)   84

9. Steve (First drink, age 12)   97

10. Lauren (First drug, age 15)   108

11. If Only I Had Known   119

WHO ARE THE PEOPLE?

The people whose stories you will be reading wrote this book. Like an editor on a newspaper, I simply made their experiences and suggestions easy to read. Nothing they said is sugar coated; so some things may shock you, scare you or make you laugh. Some events may be hard for you to believe.

Each storyteller was roughly your age, a few years younger or older, when he or she first got involved with alcohol or drugs or both. You're saying to yourself, "I'd never go that far. Not me. I'll never have a problem." That's what they said. That's what everyone thinks about alcoholism and drug addiction when he or she is drinking or drugging to be social or for a few kicks.

They're telling you what happened to them, what they wish they had known before and what they have learned, because it might be helpful to you. They are not telling you what to do. They know you will do as you please. They did.

ABOUT THE MODELS

None of the people shown in these photographs is the alcoholic, addict, friend or relative he or she portrays. The models were selected solely for their ability to convey the characters' looks, feelings and personalities.

To agree to be shown as a habitual user of drugs, part of the drug culture or a parent of a child with an addiction problem was a difficult decision for many models and their parents. To everyone who participated, thank you for giving this book its photographic life. Your pictures provide a sense of reality and make the complex world of alcohol and drugs a little bit easier to comprehend.

IT WON'T
HAPPEN TO ME

1
■
IT WON'T HAPPEN TO ME

You can't drive a car anywhere in this country until you read a driver's manual, learn the risks and rules, pass a thorough written exam and finally a supervised road test. There are no similar requirements for drinking alcohol or using other drugs, although both have as many—maybe more—hazards. As you may or may not know, alcohol *is* a drug. Whenever the word "drug" is mentioned, it refers to alcohol as well as other habit-forming drugs.

This book of case histories will be your "driver's manual" of information on drugs. By the time you finish you will have a good understanding of what it's like to be a young drinker and/or drugger.

As you read you may think, "It won't happen to me. I'm not a bit like Courtney or Martin or Gary or Melissa." It's true, we're all different. Our families, friends and backgrounds are unique. But somewhere in each chapter you'll find a little bit of your own life: a brother, an alcoholic parent, a separation, a move, a group of friends, a party, an achievement, a disappointment . . . something. These stories are not about you, but given a different set of circumstances, you could be any one of these people.

In this country one-third of the people drink pretty regularly, many abusing alcohol; one-third drink only occasionally; and one-third never drink at all. These numbers are changing rapidly. More and more adults are drinking less and less. It's pretty safe to guess that within the next ten years two-thirds are going to fall into the never-drink-at-all category.

Nonetheless, drinking and drugging still attract many young people today. Peers are often shocked when a friend turns down a drink or admits that he's never sampled pot, crack or cocaine. They gasp as if to say, "Where have you been?" That's how widespread drug use is and how "normal" teenagers view its users.

Why should you learn more than you already know about drugs? Because they're everywhere. Because there is or probably will be great pressure on you to try drugs. Because young people, including well-known sports figures and movie stars, have died from what they surely believed were harmless amounts of drugs. Because what you decide affects your health and the way your life will go, now and in the future. You, not your parents (although sometimes it doesn't feel that way), really control what you do. As you know, there's always a way to get a drink or a drug if you want it.

Sometimes you are going to have to be very strong; on other occasions you are going to need someone to talk to; and still other times you are even going to say to yourself, "Why not?" Knowing fact from fiction about drugs can make a big difference.

The facts follow each story in the sections titled You Should Know. You will learn that one out of every fifteen teens who drink becomes an alcoholic; that without meaning to, parents and other adults often "help" teenagers stay on drugs; that drinking fast can kill you. The sections called Think About focus on problems such as what to do if a close friend is overdoing it with drugs; do your parents set the best example for you; what's involved in breaking a drug habit and much more.

The stories are true. What happened to these people has happened to thousands of others. Like most kids involved with drugs today, they used more than one mind-altering drug. How much is too much? How much is too much—for you? The more you know about the power of alcohol and other drugs, the better able you will be to decide what you want to do.

2.

TERRY

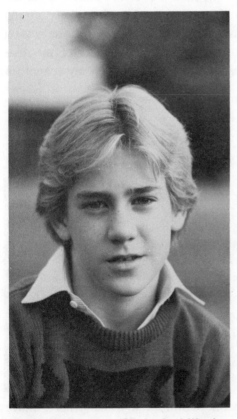

Terry, a high school freshman in Terre Haute, Indiana, ranks fifth in a class of eight hundred, is on the varsity wrestling and junior varsity soccer teams. His father is an executive with a manufacturing company; his mother is a homemaker. Like Terry, his eighteen-year-old brother did very well in school and was a fine athlete. Both boys have jobs during summer and school vacations. Theirs is a busy, happy household.

■   ■   ■

Last year I saw my brother drunk, laughing and clowning in the stands at some of the football games. He looked like he was having a great time, but he also looked silly. I was curious about how he felt, but I was afraid to ask.

My friends kept telling me drinking was terrific. I had never tried it. I felt left out. I wanted to be like everyone else. I thought if I didn't drink, people would talk about me. I was the only freshman on the wrestling team. The other guys were juniors and seniors. Same thing on the soccer team. Everyone was older than I was.

One night four of us from the wrestling team drove to watch the state competitions. An older friend of one of the senior wrestlers bought vodka for us. We mixed it with orange juice and drank screwdrivers in the car. I had one. I relaxed, I let go. I felt better about myself after that, more like them, a little older. I knew what it was all about.

During wrestling season you have to lose weight to make your weight class. My mom doesn't like it. The pressure builds up for me to cut that weight and still prove to my mom that I can keep up my grades. Sometimes I run out of energy because I eat less. She gets on me, but I don't want to give up wrestling. I like to think of myself as a jock, not a "Dexter." That's the name they use in my school for kids who are real smart.

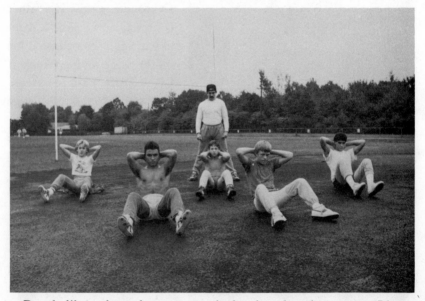

People like to hear that someone is dumb rather than smart. I have a very rough time with the wrestling team because I study before matches and go home to study after them. The other guys go out and party. They tease me, but I know my parents would have a fit if my grades started to slip. I'm always looking for ways to prove to those guys that I'm not just a student, that I'm just as cool as they are. It's hard.

The weekend after the state matches there was a school dance on Friday night. A group of us decided we would drink a little, catch a movie and head over to the dance. After school we walked to the mall and hid in the weeds behind the movie theater with some vodka, gin and Old Grand-dad that one of the boys had taken from his parents' house.

He had poured the liquor into those big vitamin bottles so we wouldn't get caught. I discovered that when you're drinking shots, if you drink them fast, you can't taste or feel them going down.

They decided to skip the movie, but I don't remember anything after we climbed out of the weeds. They told me I was screaming and falling down when we went to get a snack. When we left the restaurant, we started to walk to the dance, but I was stumbling. They yelled at me and tried to keep me on my feet.

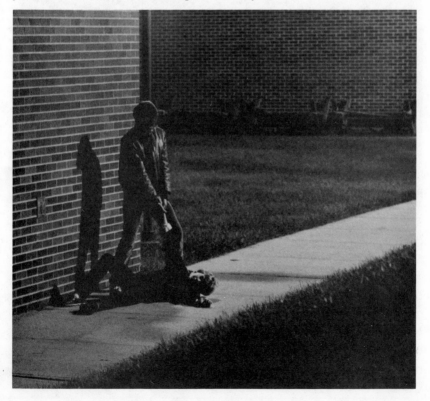

We got as far as a group of stores in the shopping mall. One of the managers heard me screaming and crying and thought it was a fight. He called the police. All the guys ran except my friend Ned. He stayed with me and got me to the back of the mall. He was drunk, too, but he knew something was wrong with me. I was out of control, throwing my arms around, crying and kicking. I'd fall down, he'd pick me up. That's what Ned tells me, anyway.

The police restrained me and drove Ned and me to the hospital. Ned says I answered the officer's questions perfectly, including reciting the alphabet and counting backward from 10 to 0. They pumped my stomach—that is not fun—to get as much alcohol out of my body as possible.

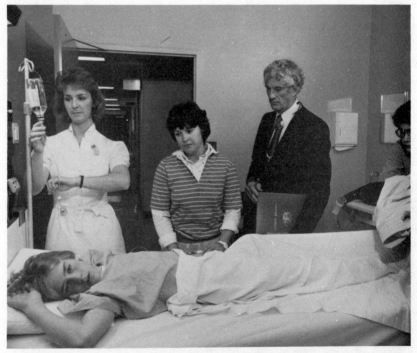

When I woke up I had a needle in my arm running up to a hanging bottle. Ned was at the end of the bed looking scared; my mom was crying. The doctor asked me: Who is the current President of the United States? I thought that was a very stupid question to ask a kid who's fifth in his class. I didn't know that he was trying to find out if my brain was functioning.

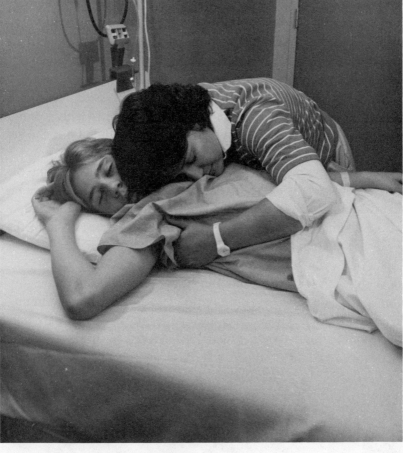

The doctor, who is our family doctor, started yelling at my mother. He gave it to her about putting too much strain on me. "Why don't you let the kid have some fun? Lay off him before you kill him." My mom just cried. I kept saying, "I'm sorry. I'm sorry." And my mom kept hugging me and saying, "I'm sorry. I'm sorry."

I have no idea how much I had to drink, but my blood alcohol content had reached .35 by the time the police brought me to the hospital. At .30 it is possible, although not usual, for someone to die. At the level I was at, it's very easy to go into a coma. Levels above .40 slow down breathing and heartbeat, and any drinker who gets to .60 is probably dead. When I heard this I knew why everyone was crying and screaming . . . and scared. I was, too.

When my father reached the hospital he started yelling at me and my mom was yelling at him. I guess they were pretty upset. My brother had never gotten into any trouble, and I think they figured I was a Dexter, that I was smart enough to stay out of trouble. But being a Dexter didn't mean I understood drinking.

I didn't know that straight shots get you drunk faster than mixed drinks. I hadn't eaten because I was trying to lose weight. I didn't know alcohol works faster on an empty stomach. I didn't mean to get that drunk. I just didn't know.

The other guys made it to the dance, and by Monday morning the whole school knew what had happened. I didn't want to go to school, but my mother forced me. In the halls the kids teased me. A couple of teachers mentioned it jokingly. For about a week I thought the world was talking about me. The incident had spread to the other schools. Everyone knew.

The guys on the team made fun of me for a real long time. My parents grounded me for two months. I had to come home immediately after practice every day, and parties on weekends were out. The first few times I went to parties I refused to drink. The kids asked why. I told them I didn't want to repeat what had happened to me.

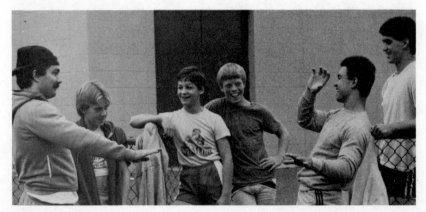

Ned and I had to go to the police station to sign an agreement to see a counselor and do community service so that our conduct and pickup would not go on record. For four weeks we washed police cars, stapled papers, cleaned up park playgrounds and washed windows at the library.

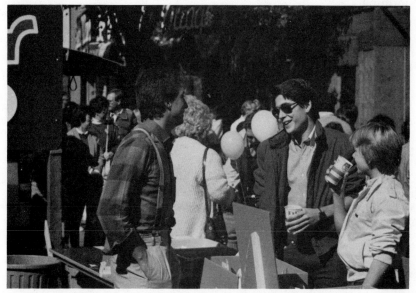

Before I go out, my parents still make me promise that I won't drink. That helps a little because it reminds me of my almost-coma. But it's not good enough. It's very hard to say no. I have a terrible time.

One of my Dexter friends doesn't drink. He doesn't have any trouble. I feel I need to give an excuse. My friend says I don't need one. I can just say No and walk away.

I try to stay away from drinking as much as possible. But just the other day I was at the fair with Ned and a bunch of guys from the soccer team. We poured wine coolers into paper cups and walked right through the fair. Nobody bothered us. I didn't have a reason not to drink. I'm the only one who remembers the night of the dance. Before the fair closed down, I had had four wine coolers. It becomes a competition to see who can drink the most.

I should know better. I might never have come out of my near-coma. After the fair I was thinking, why did I do that? What's the big deal? I have too much going for me to blow it.

YOU SHOULD KNOW

1. Before we would snort cocaine or shoot heroin, most of us would stop, at least the first time, to think about what we are doing to ourselves. Alcohol can be just as destructive and is just as habit-forming.

2. Because alcohol is socially acceptable, the drug viewed as "proper," people forget that it is as potent and deadly as cocaine, Quaaludes, angel dust and many other laboratory and street drugs.

3. The first drugs sampled by young people are usually beer and wine.

4. Surprisingly, a 12-ounce bottle of beer, a 5-ounce glass of wine and a 1½-ounce shot of whiskey have the same amount of alcohol. The only difference is the amount of water, coloring and flavorings that are added.

5. The younger a person starts drinking, the more likely it is that he will drink more heavily, drink stronger drinks and have a drinking or drug problem when he is older.

6. Most people are convinced that they will never have a problem, that they can control their drinking. Drinking starts out innocently; then suddenly a person finds he "needs" a drink, then two, then four. When a person no longer has control over his use of drugs, he is called dependent or addicted.

7. Some people seem to hold their liquor better than others. Reactions to alcohol are different and vary according to a person's body weight, body fat, amount of water in the body, point in menstrual cycle and general physical and emotional health.
   This is not a rule, but usually the same amount of alcohol will affect a smaller person more than a larger one; females, more than males.

8. Alcohol is a very simple substance that gets into the body's organs quickly, within minutes after swallowing. It goes immediately into the bloodstream and brain, changing a person's thinking and behavior. It affects the central nervous system, which includes the brain cells that send vital messages to other parts of the body.

9. The good effects of alcohol—feelings of exhilaration and relaxation—are normally produced with very small amounts. At first you feel stimulated, but as the alcohol in the bloodstream increases, it begins to work as a sedative, slowing you down. Like anesthesia used in hospitals, eventually it puts you to sleep, causes you to pass out, turns you into a medical emergency like Terry or worse.

THINK ABOUT

1. Too many people treat alcohol as if it were soda. Thirsty? Have a beer. Hot? Cool down with a gin and tonic. Cold? Warm up with a hot toddy. They drink too fast, too much, too often.

2. Being able to hold your liquor, that is, not getting wildly giddy, revoltingly sick, miserably depressed or not experiencing terrible hangovers, is dangerous because people think that the alcohol is not affecting them. Without showing, alcohol is working on the liver, heart and other body organs.

3. There are no health warnings on alcohol. Yet every package of cigarettes carries a warning label. Prescription drugs and over-the-counter pills (including aspirin) list specific dangers, correct dosage and possible side effects. Labels tell people how to use the medication properly to avoid an overdose or any harmful side effects.

4. There was probably more to Terry's drinking than simple curiosity and a desire to be like the older boys. Terry tried too hard to be good at *everything* he did, including drinking. He put himself under constant pressure to do well in school and in sports. His parents

expected only the best from him. To please parents on all levels, all the time, is asking too much of any kid.

5. "Problem" children aren't the only ones who develop unsafe habits with drugs and alcohol.

6. Drinking or drugging starts for a variety of reasons: to be liked, to have fun, to imitate parents, to appear grown-up. Preteens and teens who begin to drink and drug heavily have other explanations, as you will see in the next chapters.

3
KIMBERLY

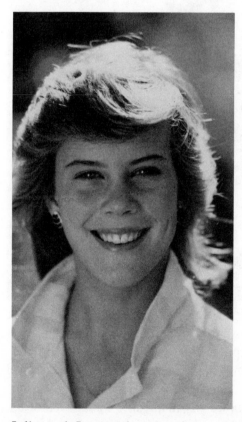

"I was one of the lucky ones," says sixteen-year-old Kimberly. "I didn't have to walk the streets or steal for my drugs and alcohol." An unhappy home was a good excuse for escaping into drugs. When she was using Kim didn't care what her peers thought. She still doesn't. Kim is very much her own person.

. . .

Daring. Crazy. Willing to try anything. That's what my mom said about me from the time I was a little girl. I'm sure I didn't think I was taking any chances in fifth grade when my friend Julie and I started eating her mother's prescription painkillers. There were bottles of them in every cabinet in Julie's house. We took a supply and refilled it whenever we needed more. They made us feel good, a little lightheaded and numb. Weird. In sixth grade Julie and I were still chewing her mother's pills.

Throughout elementary and junior high school there were four of us—Julie, Paula, Ashley and me—who drank and partied. Nobody else in the school was like us. Teachers knew, the principal knew, the other kids knew, but nobody did anything. My mom thought I was a typical kid experimenting with beer. She didn't try to stop me.

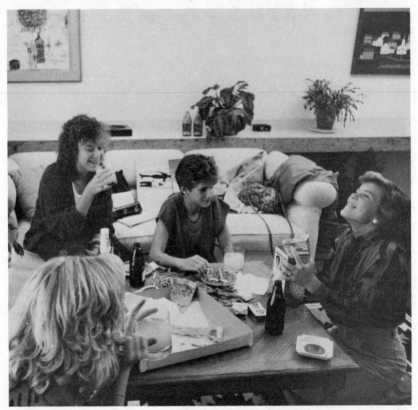

On weekends we had our own private parties. Guys who were "legal" got us anything we wanted. Julie dreamed up a drink that was wicked, a punch that I could drink by the milk carton. It barely made me high. I became known as the biggest drinker in town, but I overdid it sometimes. I spent days vomiting, lying on the bathroom floor and hugging the toilet bowl. My mom, who's a lab technician, dragged me to her hospital for tests. She and the doctors would agree that I had "that same virus again, but it's working its way out of her system."

Freshman year of high school I went downhill so fast that I never finished the term. I cut regularly to drive around and drink with my friends. My friends were truly my friends, or so I thought at the time. That's how I really got hooked. Beginning with Julie, my friends gave me booze and drugs: gin, vodka, beer, speed, acid, coke, pot. I never had to pay. It was a free ride for me all the way down the road.

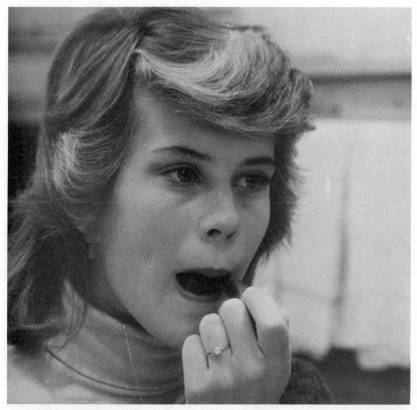

I became known as speed queen by the kids in school. They called me slut and other things, but I didn't care. I did care enough about myself to avoid getting run down. So many addicts don't care about themselves. They don't take showers; they don't eat. No matter what happened I took a shower and spent a half-hour doing my hair and makeup before I went out to do my drugs.

The only other thing I cared about was getting caught. Cops. Parents. I was paranoid and looked over my shoulder constantly. I lied to my parents, snuck out of my room every night and ran away about every other week. I was never very close to my mother, and the times we were getting along, my stepfather would get jealous and start arguing with her and picking on me. It wasn't very pleasant. Even though I was only fifteen, I ran away to upset them.

My older friends had apartments and were glad to have me. Sometimes I stayed with them for a week, once two weeks. I wanted my independence. I didn't want to pedal my bike or have my mother drive me whenever I wanted to go out. I liked staying with friends: No adult telling me what to do and when to do it. But I always went back home.

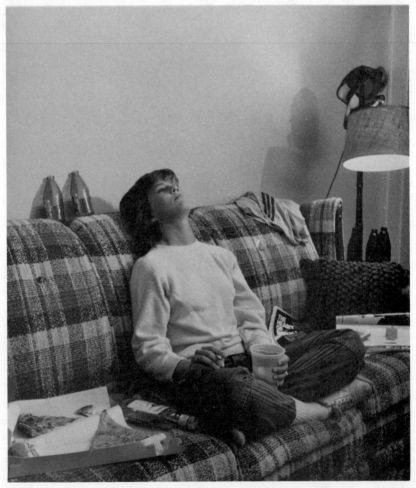

The last time I took off it was with a guy I had *just met* at Ashley's house. I sat in his apartment for two days thinking about what I was

doing. I had lost my self-respect and my morals. I had no responsibilities: I stopped going to school or helping out at home. I didn't
feel guilty because I had no feelings other than I want this drug; I
need it now. I had no control over myself. Alcohol and drugs con-
trolled me. I felt cold. I had no feelings for anyone. I didn't know a
person could feel that way.

I must have had that little something left in me that I needed. I
called my mother and told her I was coming home. I guess she didn't
believe me. When I got home no one was there. I was pretty sure my
mom had filed a runaway report on me. I called the police to tell
them that I was back. It certainly wasn't the first time she had
reported me missing.

Our school keeps a list of kids they know or suspect have a drug
problem. They were not surprised to hear from my mother. The
drug counselor and principal found help for me. I was put into a full-
time rehabilitation program immediately. That was March of my
freshman year.

During group therapy I was angry and talked only about the kids
who did drugs and always seemed to be fine. There was one guy at
school who was captain of the basketball team, number one on the
boys' track team, on the honor roll. Tim could drink, get stoned and
still perform perfectly. Adults had no idea. And if you mentioned it,
people were horrified: "Oh, no, not Tim."

I couldn't understand: Why couldn't I be like Tim or Julie or
Ashley? I complained about my older friends who had their own
cars, their own apartments, everything they wanted and drank and
were stoned daily. How could they do it? I asked every time it was
my turn to speak. I did not listen when other people talked about
their problems. I sulked and tuned out. I resented everybody in and
out of that place.

Within a couple of months it was clear that I was making no
progress. My mother moved me to a much stricter program run by
nuns for the summer. We lived in bungalows in the middle of the
Michigan woods. You had to get up at six in the morning, make your
bed, get to classes. They didn't fool around. If you weren't doing
well in your courses, you were sent to a study hall from seven to
eleven at night. There were group therapy meetings and lectures on
drugs and living.

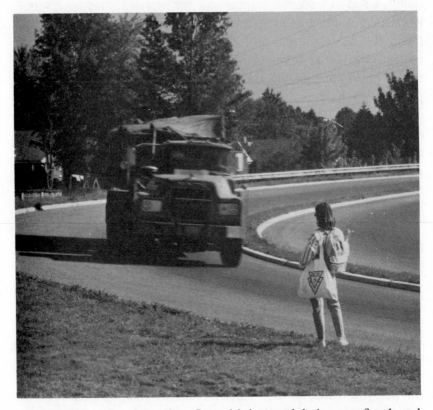

I couldn't take the rules. I couldn't stand being confined and ordered around. I ran away twice. The first time I called my mother, who refused to come for me. She called the school and was told that if I wanted to come back to the program I would find a way. I dragged myself back because I didn't know where to go or what else to do. I stayed until I decided I could stay straight on my own.

Two weeks later I hitchhiked home. My mother was surprised to see me and not too sure I could manage by myself. I saw a counselor every Tuesday and Thursday and went to Alcoholics Anonymous (AA) meetings for over a year, but I was able to start school in the fall with my class.

It was time, I told myself, to do something good for me. I wanted to be on the running team, but my school has a strict point policy and because I had missed half of my freshman year I did not have the required points. The counselor went to the coach in charge and then to the principal to convince them to make an exception.

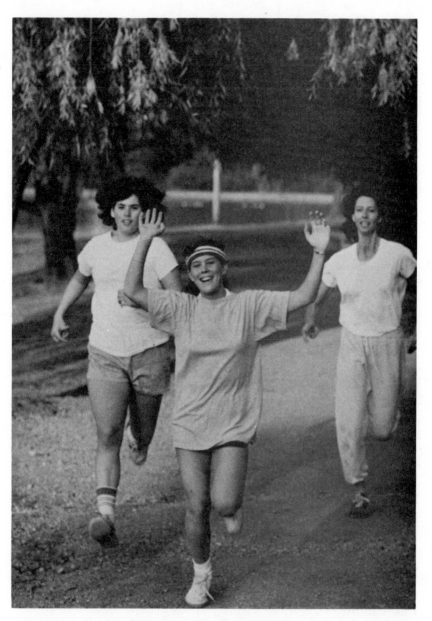

Last year (sophomore year) I was second-best cross-country run-
ner in the school and on the honor roll. I have lots of new friends.
I've heard that the guys I used to hang around with have lost their
apartments and cars. Somebody told me they've turned into real
scumbags.

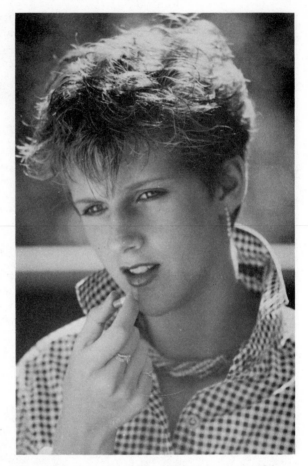

Julie is still using. So are Paula and Ashley. They have been able to keep up their grades. Paula fights more with her parents and Ashley has started sleeping with different guys. Their problems are getting bigger, but they haven't been done in like I was . . . yet.

I could not control myself. Once I had a little I had to keep going. I had to do more and more and more. My old friends say that they can do without it. I couldn't. Maybe they are different from me and what I have in my body, what my body needs.

I don't want to go back to where I was. I'm glad it's over. My friends know that I've changed. They don't come over to me with drinks or try to get me to use drugs. They drink in front of me, but it doesn't bother me. I'm the girl who could knock off a case of beer by herself!

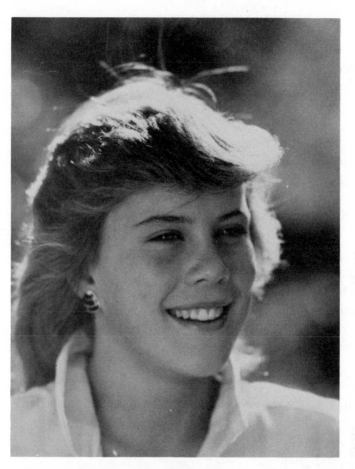

I'm still wild and crazy. I'll swing from a rope over a river when no one else will. I love fast cars and dangerous amusement park rides. I haven't lost my spirit. But I can never forget that I'm an alcoholic and a drug addict. I'm sixteen. I won't even be able to have a glass of champagne at my own wedding.

YOU SHOULD KNOW

1. Alcoholism is a disease. Continued and increased drinking creates problems that only get worse and that almost always are harmful to the individual and/or the people around her, especially family and friends.

2. Some people choose to abuse alcohol and other drugs but can stop at will. Others have the tendency to become addicted, and stopping, even when they want to, is extremely difficult. Addiction is a real physical need. The craving becomes stronger if the person is unhappy or having other emotional problems.

3. Most people don't know they have this disease until it's too late. Stopping and staying stopped can be learned, but alcoholism cannot be erased. Once an alcoholic, always an alcoholic. Unlike poison ivy or pneumonia, alcoholism does not disappear after treatment. One sip for a recovered alcoholic even after years "on the wagon" is too much. She will react to alcohol as if she had been drinking last night.

4. If you were asked to describe an alcoholic, your image might be something like this: a man lying prone in the street with an empty pint of booze clutched in his hand. He needs a shave and a two-hour soaking in a soapy tub. His clothes are filthy, and he doesn't look as if he would be very smart.

The fact is that very few of the 10 million known (admitted) alcoholics in this country are bums. Most alcoholics have homes, families and jobs. Many are famous writers, athletes, rock stars and movie personalities.

5. Kimberly is one of the young problem drinkers who was an alcoholic before she was old enough to drive. She is not unusual. Studies indicate that there are almost 3½ million teenage alcoholics and another 4 million young people between the ages of twelve and seventeen who use drugs regularly.

6. Alcoholics Anonymous (AA) is a group of men, women and

young people who had or have a drinking problem and who are committed to staying sober. They meet regularly to support each other by discussing their individual experiences and offering encouragement to those who are trying to stop or stay stopped. Members know what this illness is like and explain how AA can help a person recover from alcoholism. AA, founded in 1935, is the most successful program for alcoholics and has many, many teenage members.

7. Narcotics Anonymous (NA), which concentrates on stopping addiction to drugs other than alcohol, operates the same as AA, with local chapters in most cities throughout the country that hold daily and nightly meetings. Members are identified by first names only; there are no educational or age requirements and no fees for either group.

The front section of most phone books lists special services available for dealing with drug and alcohol problems. Also check the White Pages under the group or organization name.

THINK ABOUT

1. We mostly think of an alcoholic as someone who has twenty or thirty years of drinking under his or her belt. We don't think of a fourteen-year-old girl or a twelve-year-old boy. We don't think of our best friend as being addicted to alcohol or amphetamines (stimulants). We think instead that she's too young; she's too smart. Kimberly thought that way too.

2. Drinking isn't bad in the same sense that robbing a bank is bad. Rather, drinking is an illness for some people. They don't know alcohol is damaging their physical and mental health until they are in trouble. With each drinking episode for the alcoholic, the reaction is more serious.

3. Running away repeatedly had no good or bad effect on Kim's addiction. There is no help "out there," only deeper problems and a harder life.

4. Someone can be a freeloader just so long—generally not as long as Kim—before she must scrape together the money to buy her own drugs and alcohol.

5. Kim believed, "My friends were truly my friends." Kim really needed a friend who discouraged her drinking, a caring friend who understood how hard it is to kick a drug and alcohol habit.

6. This special friend would have asked Kim to get help and kept after her until she did. The friend would have said, "Why are you doing this to yourself?" She would have told Kim that she cared and was worried about her. The friend Kim needed would have said, "I love you. You must do something to stop."

7. When a person is into drugs as deeply as Kim, pressure to find help could save his or her life.

4.

MARTIN

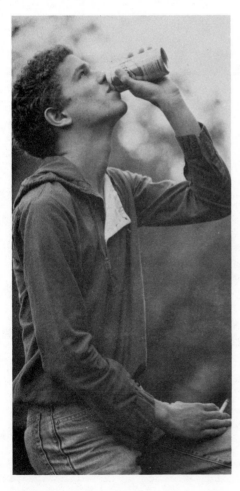

Martin was born in Des Moines, Iowa, the oldest of five children. The family moved three times by the time he graduated from high school. Martin had no restrictions and no guidance from his parents. Until he went for help for his father, the only thing he knew about alcohol was that "beer was bad."

■ ■ ■

We moved to White Plains, New York, because my dad got a great job selling television time for commercials. I was nine years old, in the fourth grade. To me, everyone acted, talked and dressed differently, but I joined Little League and tried very hard to make new friends. In no time I belonged and was happy.

In the spring of sixth grade my class took a trip to Washington, D.C. When I came home there was a big fat "Sold" sign in front of our house. I thought it was a mistake. I didn't want to move. I loved my school and my friends. We were excited about being in junior high and talked about how we were going to be in the same classes. I was so disappointed that I did not speak to my mother or father for one whole month.

This time we moved to a tiny country town in upstate New York with one kid my age within walking distance and nothing—I mean nothing—to do unless you're into planting corn and milking cows. Zero. At least not after what I had been used to in bustling White Plains, which is real close to New York City. There we were dating; here, the boys thought girls were gross. What a bunch of stupid, nowhere kids.

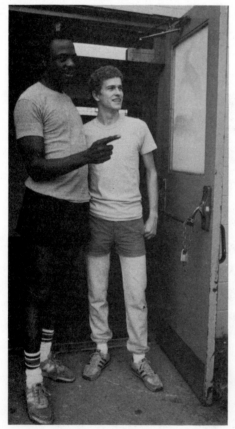

This is where I'm going to spend the rest of my life? I hated it, but I was willing to try. Sports failed me. The only decent team the school had was basketball. I was too short to be any good. So I wrote off sports except for track, whose biggest and only fans were the coach and me. We got into it, studying the curves, looking over the competition. He thought I had a great running future. I was way ahead of the kids my age academically. There didn't seem to be any way for me to be like them.

My father had a two-hour drive to his new job. You didn't have to be a genius to figure that he didn't get a promotion: The drive, the town and the tiny, shabby house we lived in were proof of that. My father left at six-thirty in the morning; got home about nine or nine-thirty at night, stormed around, then sat on the couch and drank. I stayed away from him as much as possible because of his terrible rages.

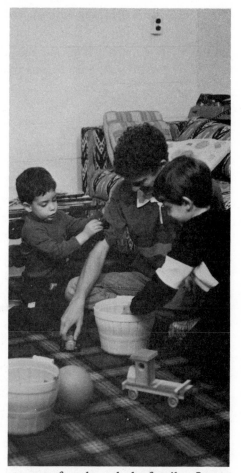

I helped my mother with my sisters and brothers, especially the youngest ones. I fed them, dressed them, bathed them and played with them. I mowed the grass, took care of the yard and baby-sat to bring home extra money. I did a lot of what my father should have been doing.

Ron, my best White Plains friend, was moving to Chicago, and his parents threw a big, fancy going-away party for the whole family. I was excited to go back to see everybody. I wasn't sure what to wear and was too embarrassed to ask.

My friend's mother was in a long slinky dress, the other women had lots of jewelry and party clothes and the men were in suits. The guys had on sports jackets and ties; some of my old friends were wearing suits. I felt like one of the nowhere kids in my pressed jeans and shirt. I was very self-conscious.

Ron got champagne and screwdrivers from somebody and gave them to us. I drank whatever was put in my hand. I forgot about my clothes. I loosened up and fit in—tight!—with my old gang. It was great.

At that party I discovered the key to my crummy hick town. From then on I started drinking with the guys. What else was there to do in seventh grade? That's what we did most weekends. Nothing else mattered. For me it wiped out the differences. I drank with these guys for years, needing more and more beer to get high.

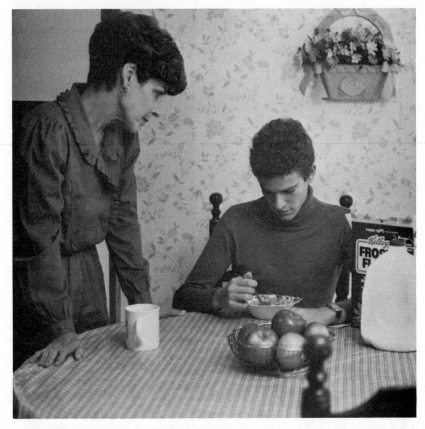

Weekends when my father was traveling on business were especially wild. I didn't get caught until freshman year. I had consumed two six-packs of beer and walked clumsily into the kitchen. It was midnight and my mother would not let me go to bed. At my fifth bowl of Frosted Flakes, she got up her nerve. "You've been drinking, haven't you?" I told her I didn't want to talk and dragged myself upstairs.

The next morning she was on me again. "Why do you drink?"

"I like it. It tastes good. It's fun. You know, Mom, a real good time?"

"Well, are you ever going to do it again?" she asked.

"You betcha." I laughed.

"Your father's going to have to deal with this."

I was petrified. When he got home from his trip, I waited and waited for him to yell. He didn't mention it, my mother didn't say another word and I certainly wasn't going to bring it up.

I didn't worry about becoming an alcoholic because I didn't know what alcoholism was. I didn't know that was my father's problem or the reason we kept moving and having money, then not having money. I knew one thing: I didn't want to be around the house.

I left for school early in the morning and stayed out until I was pretty sure my mother would be asleep; my father, passed out. When I was home, I mouthed off constantly: I told my parents that I didn't like them, that I thought they were nuts. I wanted to know why I couldn't have friends over, why we never went out to dinner.

"I think you have some serious mental problems," my mom told me during my sophomore year. "I want you to see a counselor."

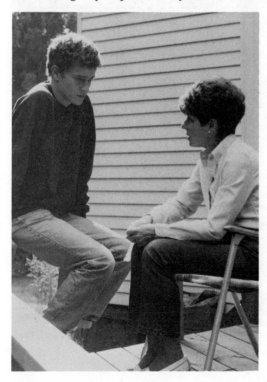

After four months of treatment, the counselor asked to see the whole family.

That was one crazy scene, focusing on the fact that my mother was missing money. I wasn't stealing, but my mother thought I was. I thought it must be one of my younger brothers or sisters. They screamed and yelled and accused me. After the session the whole family was convinced I was guilty. I started to cry and hated myself for being so weak.

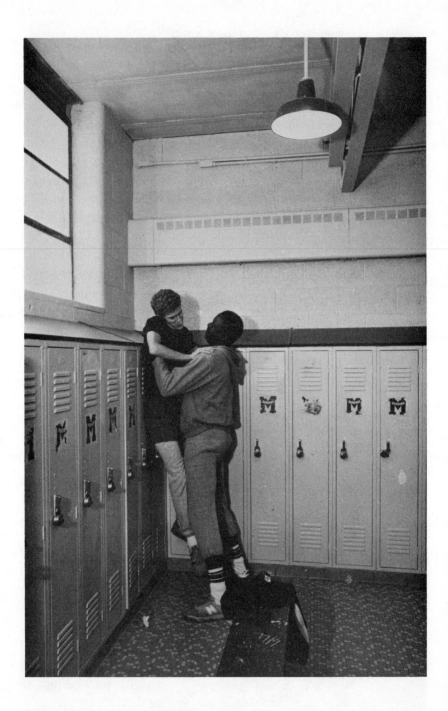

Here I had been playing daddy, doing the yard work, helping out, and no one cared. Neither did I. I quit track. The coach was furious. He picked me up and threw me against the lockers. "You're going to be a quitter the rest of your life," he shouted. That's when I started drinking and smoking pot during the week as well as on weekends. I was grouchy and sullen for the rest of high school.

I don't think my mother wanted to know what I was doing. She wanted to believe that I had stopped after the night she caught me in ninth grade. My father was more than she could handle. Senior year she told me we had to talk, that she had something distressing and very important to tell me. "Your father's an alcoholic," she said with big tears running down her face.

"What's that?" I asked innocently. I didn't see any great need for tears.

I went to Alateen to learn about my father's illness. There I found out that I had a fifty-fifty chance or better of becoming an alcoholic if

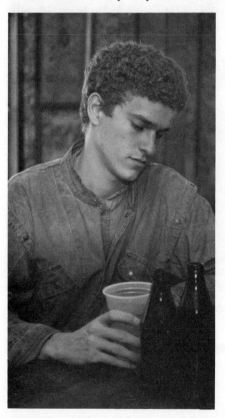

I drank. That scared me a little, but not enough to stop me. The way I saw it, I was having a good time.

Because I was a good student I could drink, smoke pot and still sail through school. I did very well on my college boards and was set to go off to college in the fall following graduation. I was happy because that meant I would be out of the house permanently. During that summer my father lost his job and with it, my college tuition. The house had to be sold, and the family was moving again.

Not me. The same day I heard the news, I packed my stuff and rented a room. I worked for a printer and drank. All the time. At this point I could drink a lot and not appear drunk. After a year on printing presses and barstools, I knew I was drinking too much and not really having fun. I tried to stop, but I was drinking compulsively.

At first I could stop for a week, but then I couldn't stop for one day. Not one single day! I wanted to stop so badly. I told myself: not today, not a drop. By noon I couldn't stand it. I raced to the nearest bar. There was nothing to do but keep drinking. With all I knew by then about my father and alcoholism from Alateen, I still didn't think I had a problem.

Many nights I could not drive home from the bar or a "friend's" house. The guys I drank with weren't my friends. I know that today. They were just people to sit with while I guzzled beer and got smashed. I don't think I knew anyone's last name.

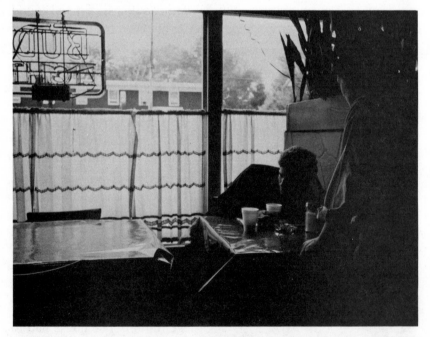

Before I tried to drive, I would drink cups and cups of black coffee. I would go outside and take deep breaths, and if I was in awful shape I would find someone's hose and douse myself with cold water. In the car I shouted, usually pretty much the same thing: "You're doing great. That's a boy. Terrific. Hug that yellow line. Steady, down the center."

My driving was a joke. Luckily I survived seeing cars that weren't there, swerving to miss cars that were. Thank God for that yellow line.

One night I got picked up for drunk driving. I fell down when the cop asked me to walk my beloved yellow line. I spent the night in jail shivering in my hosed-down clothes. I understood why my mother had cried so hard when she told me about my father. I was an alcoholic, too. The next night I went to an AA meeting instead of a bar.

A year later in an AA meeting I was listening to a guy tell how he stole to support his addiction. It came to me—my younger brothers and sisters had not been stealing from my mother. My father was!

YOU SHOULD KNOW

1. A person doesn't wake up one morning and say to himself, "Aha. I'm going to be a heavy drinker." For those with alcohol problems, the course of events is slow and sneaky. Without them being aware of it, their drinking increases until it is out of control.

2. It is not necessary to drink "hard liquor" such as vodka, rye or bourbon to become an alcoholic. The guy who knocks off a six-pack of beer or a bottle of wine every other night is as likely to have a chronic problem as the gal who sips her father's Scotch every day after school.

3. People who get plastered *only* on weekends, let's say, or just Thursday nights when their parents are out, have a habit that's as dangerous as those who drink daily.

4. The person who drinks once a month,even if he has *only one* drink, then picks fights or becomes a loudmouth, rips off his clothes or punches out someone, has a serious problem, too. He should not drink. It is not necessarily the quantity but rather how the body and brain react.

5. Frequent drinkers begin to build up a physical resistance called tolerance to this drug. As tolerance increases, the drinker requires greater quantities of alcohol to produce a "buzz," to have a good time, to strip away his inhibitions or to think he feels better about himself.

6. A responsible drinker, your average drinker, would get nauseous or pass out, on the amount of liquor an alcoholic with high tolerance must consume to make him feel "normal."

7. If your tolerance is built up for beer, let's say, it will also be high for other alcoholic beverages.

8. Coffee, fresh air and cold showers may make the drinker feel wide

awake, but they do not make him sober. It takes about two hours for the body to eliminate one ounce of alcohol, the amount in an average drink. In other words, time is the only way to sober up and sleeping is probably the best way to pass that time.

The body needs about 15½ hours (more than half a day) to burn up the alcohol in a six-pack of beer, longer if you weigh less than 120 pounds, slightly less time if you weigh more.

9. Alateen is a group of teenagers who meet to help each other find ways to cope with the problems of living with an alcoholic parent. Like AA, the program helps teens feel less alone and less awkward because of a drinking parent. It's excellent support when the going is rough at home, because Alateen members live or have lived with many of the same troubles, pain and shame. Al-Anon offers the same assistance to husbands and wives of alcoholics.

If Alateen is not listed in the phone book, called Alcoholics Anonymous or your local Alcohol Information Center to locate the nearest Alateen chapter.

THINK ABOUT

1. Moving is always upsetting. Moving means starting over. Most people have a difficult time. Martin had other choices when he moved upstate. He could have taken up photography, tried working on one of the farms or devoted himself to a noncompetitive sport such as swimming or weight lifting.

2. Placing the blame for excessive drinking or drugging elsewhere is an easy out: on parents for moving, for having a baby when you think they're too old, for paying more attention to their jobs than they do to you, for divorcing or for being too strict or too lenient.

The drinker can think his teachers are responsible for his problems because they flunked him or the coach because he kept him off the team. But the real fault belongs to the drinker or drugger. He alone made the decision to get involved. No one twisted his arm or forced open his mouth.

3. Parents often have trouble discussing difficult subjects. Many parents shy way from anything more than a passing comment about death, sexual abuse, sex and drugs. This doesn't mean they don't understand or don't care.

Avoiding the issue is likely to happen if, as in the case of Martin's father, the parent is an abuser. Martin's dad was smart enough to realize that to forbid Martin to drink would be hypocritical.

4. Even a person who understands alcoholism, as Martin finally did, finds it hard to admit his own problem. Addicts make excuses, rationalize and deny their problem. They tell others that they don't need drugs; they tell themselves that they can stop whenever they want. They think this way until they try.

5. If any of the guys Martin drank with were real friends, they would have cautioned him not to drive and would have driven him home or put him up for the night.

6. Martin's drinking, like that of any other alcoholic, finally caught up with him. For almost all who are addicted, the thrill of what they're doing isn't there anymore.

5

■

SHEILA

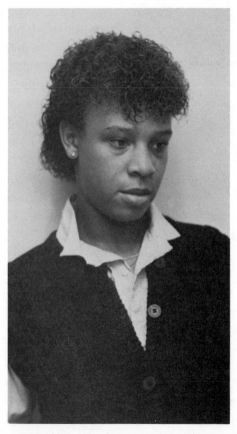

People thought Sheila was always in control. Her practical, down-to-earth manner fooled everyone. Sheila grew up in the suburbs of Providence, Rhode Island. Her mother's a first-grade teacher, her father is not alive. In spite of firsthand knowledge, "I became my worst fear—an alcoholic," she says with a look of disbelief.

■   ■   ■

I remember my first drink. I was not quite nine years old. My uncle gave me champagne at his wedding. It was delicious. I felt wonderful. I was very excited; my mother was very annoyed. For years my role was to be the "good" kid. I took care of my sister and brother by cooking and cleaning after school. I'm five years older

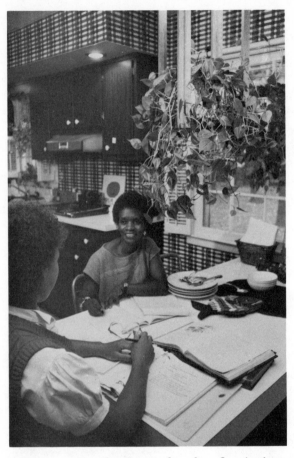

than my sister and three years older than my brother. They looked up to me. So did my mother. I was her star and I desperately wanted her approval.

I excelled in school and was on the academic fast track in junior high and high school. Because studying came easily to me, I had time to participate in student government, be on the debate team and in drama club. I was an over-achiever, very serious about my responsibilities and very, very fat: I was five feet five inches tall and weighed 170 pounds all through junior high.

I ran around with the brainy, nerdy types at school who readily accepted me, yet I always felt like a misfit. My friends were so straight; most of them did not drink. I was probably the straightest of the group.

My father died of cirrhosis of the liver when I was eleven years old, but his death certificate read: "Cause of Death: Heart Failure." He had been an active alcoholic throughout my growing years. I caught on when I was about eight, after I discovered empty bottles of vodka hidden in strange places around the house. I hated the times he beat my mother and I hated the nights, most nights, when they screamed downstairs. My younger sister crawled into my bed regularly for comfort. I promised myself I would never drink.

I was very self-righteous and immovable on the subject. But there was another side of me that was completely fascinated with alcohol. When I was a child, our family parties were very rowdy. There were large parties with lots of drinking and dancing, lots of excitement and lots of glamour that drew me in.

About a year after my father died, I dipped into the liquor cabinet after our family Thanksgiving dinner, which was more like a party in our house. I filled a water glass two-thirds with rum. I chugged it, ran upstairs to my room and lay down on my bed to see what would happen. The bed spun, just like the beaters on one of those hand mixers. I thought it was great. I didn't think it was scary. I liked the feeling.

For years, I drank alone in my bedroom whenever I could sneak a beer or pour some rum or vodka without my mother noticing. Between what I could take from my house and the liquor I stole from baby-sitting jobs, I managed to drink four or five nights a week.

My mother had put the fear of God in me about "drugs," although she and my father had Valium for breakfast. Hers was washed down with orange juice, his with a glass of Scotch. After Dad died, my mother scared me and, as they got older, my brother and sister, by warning us that alcoholism might be hereditary. I was truly afraid.

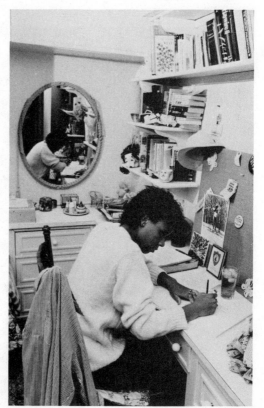

Everything I saw written about alcoholism I read with the hope of learning something new, but nothing seemed to apply to me.

In the privacy of my bedroom, drinking felt good. I had also begun to see what alcohol could do for me. It made me feel thinner, and changed how I viewed myself. I definitely liked that.

By my last two years of high school, when my friends were drinking publicly, I could drink everyone under the table including some of the guys. I had an enormous capacity. That proved very dangerous and misleading, because I felt that if I could hold my liquor I was not going to have a problem. I could not become an alcoholic like my father. However, whenever there was booze around, I drank. I drank greater and greater quantities.

In spite of my heavy drinking, I started to lose more weight. Several of my girlfriends taught me how to vomit everything I had eaten. We would go out, stuff ourselves, then go into a bathroom and force ourselves to throw up. Finally I had lost enough weight—mind you, I wasn't skinny by any stretch of the imagination—to feel a little better about myself. Guys were beginning to notice me. My social life improved.

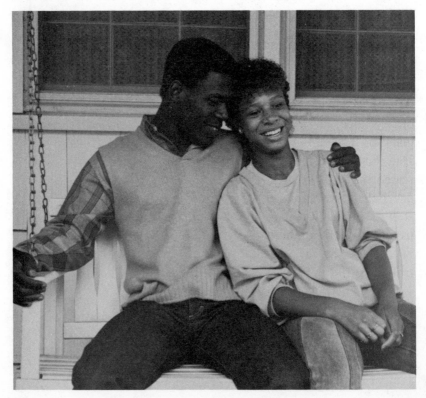

I dated Larry exclusively during my junior year and part of my senior year. Larry was not interested in alcohol because his father had a problem like mine had had. I was disappointed when he always refused to drink. I used pot and hash to control my drinking when we were together. At parties I would sneak away from him to get a drink. If there was no booze at a party, I was not happy. If there was no liquor in a house where I baby-sat, I stopped working for that family. I began to realize that drinking was becoming too important.

I have a lot of memories of not-right, not-normal drinking experiences. Like getting my hands on a bottle of gin and making the drinks so strong none of my friends could drink them, but they were okay for me. Or knocking off a whole bottle of Scotch by myself.

I remained very serious about school. I still wanted my mother's approval. I felt she would love me more if I got good grades. So I didn't drink every night. And I didn't drink every weekend. I reminded myself to watch it. I told myself I would stop when I thought I was drinking too much.

Larry kept my drinking in check until we broke up halfway through senior year. I felt alone and rejected, but I had a good excuse for drinking myself to sleep every night. I was frightened by what I was doing, but I could not stop. Now my drinking had become

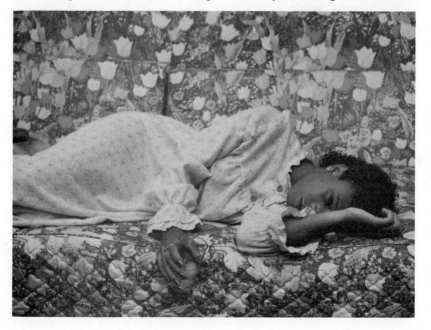

something that even I could clearly label alcoholic.

My whole life, senior year being no exception, people thought I had it together. I, on the other hand, was terrified at all times that anyone who got past my exterior would be able to look inside and see that I was crazy. I had the outside trappings that said I was together. I had tremendous school achievements. In that respect I was like my father. He had been very successful. To the world, since I did not drink during the day, I was sober and perfect.

I would start about eight at night behind the closed door of my bedroom and polish off about a third of a bottle of vodka. Drinking had lost its charm. It had been a long, long time since the bed had spun. When I drank, I felt as if I were in a coma. Like being in a wet, dark tunnel looking out into nothing. I wanted someone to notice, but no one did.

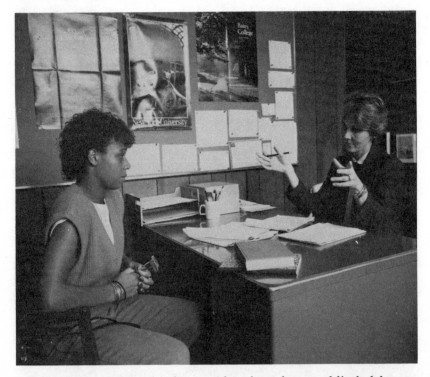

I went to see the school counselor, but she was blinded by my outstanding school record and my extracurricular activities. On top of that I thoroughly confused her by telling her I thought I had a problem, which I hastily followed by giving her all the reasons that such a thing was not possible. She believed the latter, thinking I only needed someone who would listen, and told me to stop by anytime I felt like chatting.

My mother, who must have noticed that I was becoming more and more depressed, ignored me. She didn't seem to care that I wasn't coming out of my room at night or wasn't helping around the house and had stopped talking to my brother and sister. She probably popped another Valium, closed her own door and prepared her lesson plans for the next day.

One night a week before graduation she could not ignore what was happening to me. In the middle of the night, drunk out of my mind, sobbing about Larry, I slammed my hand into the hall mirror at the top of the stairs. I became aware of what was happening as thousands of slivers of mirror grazed my hand and hit my feet. I remember my mother shouting about Alcoholics Anonymous and telling me I would have to get out of the house. I was busy examining my blood and looking at a face I didn't recognize.

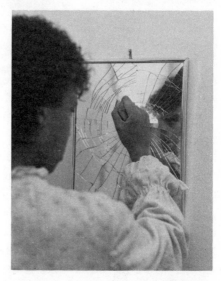

A few mornings later I woke up in my bed, which was soaked with urine. I could not remember how I got there. I had never been so bad that I didn't wake up to go to the bathroom. I thought of my father— dead. I didn't want my life to end. I called my aunt. "I'm in trouble and you have to take me seriously," I told her. She talked to my mother.

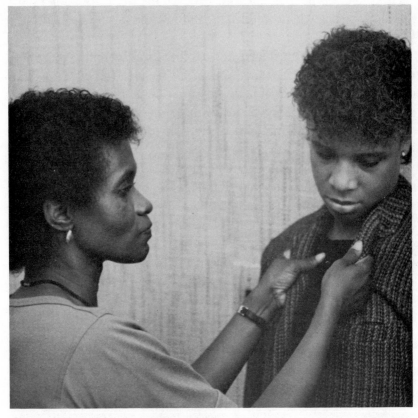

My mother was miserable and furious at the same time. She insisted I go to a rehabilitation center. When she dropped me off, she let the entire center know her true feelings. She pulled on my jacket and shouted hysterically, "You're not my daughter. I have given you the best and you turned into him [meaning my father]. I don't ever want to see you again." She left me there with no kiss, no good luck, no place to go home to, nothing. It was the fulfillment of my worst fear: if I wasn't a perfect child, I wasn't going to be loved. My mother wrote me off. It was years before I regained her love and respect.

As in school, I was the perfect rehab person. I was so busy doing what was expected of me that I never accepted the fact that I was an alcoholic. I was too young. I was a girl. I was too smart. After six weeks of doing exactly as I was told, I was released. I couldn't go home, so I went to my aunt's and called my friend Cass.

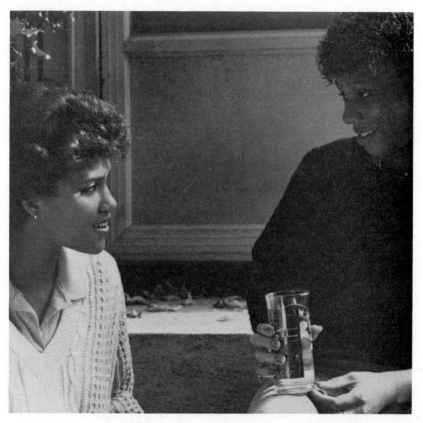

I felt great. I felt like I could drink. I did. And I couldn't. I could not stay away from alcohol. I could not stay stopped. Since then I have spent over a year in clinics, a year with special alcoholism counselors and two years going four times a week to AA meetings.

Addiction says to me, "Try it again. Go ahead." That's why I still go to meetings—to remind myself that I'd have to be crazy to drink again.

YOU SHOULD KNOW

1. Alcoholism is a sickness that ranks up there with heart disease and cancer. It's lethal, but society does not accept alcohol as a killer. Sheila's father died because alcohol rotted his liver. Doctors who completely understand the damaging effects of alcohol on the body hide the truth by lying on the death certificate so the family is not embarrassed.

2. Over years of drinking, if it is not treated, alcoholism can cause permanent liver damage, brain damage, nerve damage, heart problems, cancer of many of the body's organs, lower resistance to disease and an endless list of emotional problems.

3. Roughly 1 out of every 15 teens who drink will become an alcoholic; 1 out of every 4 will get into some kind of trouble. If you understand the risks, your chances are reduced because you can approach the drug alcohol the way it should be approached—cautiously.

4. Once you become addicted—once you cross the invisible line— you will always be addicted. The snag is that there is no way of knowing when you're approaching the line.

5. One clue for possible addiction is the ability to drink more and more. Increased tolerance is a warning signal. So is having bad feelings about drinking experiences.

6. We don't know exactly what role heredity plays, but some factors are fairly clear: More than half of today's alcoholics had at least one alcoholic parent, grandparent or close blood relative. And children whose biological parents are alcoholic are *four times* more likely to become alcoholics themselves than are children of nonalcoholics.

7. Having a close relative who is alcoholic, even if a recovered alcoholic, puts you in the high-risk category, meaning you have a greater chance of becoming an alcoholic than someone whose parents have

no problems with drinking.

Other high-risk people include American Indians and those who live with parents who choose not to drink for moral rather than medical reasons. Children who are abused by their parents are also considered high risks.

8. Alcohol is very fattening. It's made from sugars such as sugar cane, molasses and honey, and different starches such as wheat and other grains. So the calorie count is high in most drinks. A 12-ounce beer averages between 100 and 150 calories. Diet books alert readers to the "empty calories" in alcohol and warn that heavy drinking can lead to obesity.

THINK ABOUT

1. Thoughts and feelings about drinking get mixed up easily. In Sheila's case, she hated alcohol because her father's drinking caused friction in the house, but family parties were festive, rowdy and exciting in large part because of the drinking that took place. She had wonderful memories of family gatherings.

2. If parents are habitual pill poppers, as Sheila's mom and dad were—and the pills can merely be aspirin—they're teaching dependency on a chemical without realizing it. Excessive use of tranquilizers and pills of any sort, unless they are medically required, is a behavior pattern to note, but not copy.

3. If you are in a high-risk group because of alcoholism in the family, it's a good idea to hold off any experimenting with alcohol until you are older, more mature and have better emotional security to handle problems. At that point a person is less likely to fall into alcohol's traps.

4. There is not a simple reason that Sheila became an alcoholic. A number of factors work together and against any young person who drinks. There are certain times during which you can be propelled

into dangerous drinking habits more easily than others.

You will be more susceptible to the false good feelings alcohol sometimes produces if you are doing poorly in school, have lost a boyfriend or girlfriend, if your parents are separating or divorcing, if someone close to you has died, if you have lost a ball game or a part in the school play, if your parents have reduced your freedom or "dumped" on your friends. In other words, the times you're feeling low for whatever reason are not good ones for drinking.

5. Liquor doesn't work very well or very long as a camouflage. It will never make acne or freckles disappear or a lisp go silent, or turn a limp into a smooth, sexy walk. It can't change the fact that you're adopted, your mother's an alcoholic or your parents are divorced.

6

COURTNEY

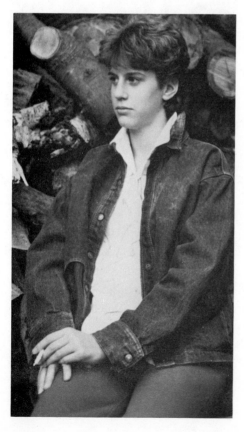

Courtney spent three days in a locked mental ward. It took her three years to straighten out her brain after a five-year bout with alcohol and pot. Courtney's family is especially loving, religious and well educated. Courtney lived in Cambridge, Massachusetts, with her parents, who would be considered very light social drinkers.

■　　■　　■

When I was very young I thought a lot about who I wanted to be when I grew up. I saw myself as being an important adult. I wanted to be someone very special.

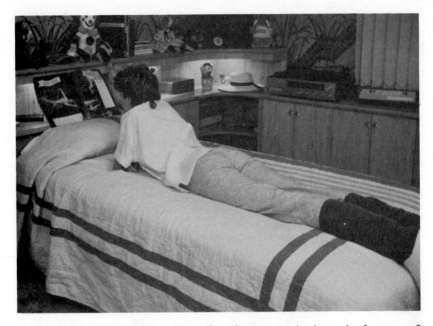

By eighth grade I shot up to five feet seven inches. At fourteen I towered over every boy and girl in my class. At parties no one danced with me. The boys wouldn't even stand near me; they teased me from across the room: "Hey, Court, how are things at the foul line?" "Is the air really thinner up there?" "Bet you don't need a ladder to paint the ceiling." Since the girls were into the boys, they ignored me, too. I felt alone in school and out.

I considered joining the circus. They must have use for a very tall person, I told myself. I wasn't brave enough to leave home. I loved my parents and could not hurt them that way. I started spending time with Jerry, the boy next door. He was a few years older and a lot taller than the boys in my class, so he thought I was okay.

One afternoon in the park Jerry convinced me to smoke a joint. He really pressured me. So I did it. I started laughing, then I started feeling funny. I only remember bits and pieces of what happened. My legs felt strange; I couldn't walk. I remember pouring water over my head, but I don't remember how I got home.

It was rocky getting into pot. The first few times I tried it, I got frightened and would hang on to Jerry. Grab him. Dig my nails into his skin. After I adjusted to it I loved it because it was predictable for me. I became a pothead.

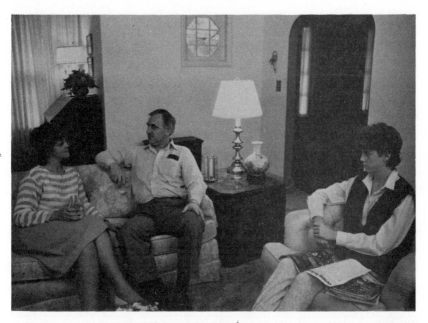

It was a good high; I felt protected and untouchable by the kids in my class. I was happy when I was stoned. I also liked the idea of pot because it was something my parents did not do; it was kind of underground, while drinking was more acceptable to them. Drinking was something parents did. Kids smoked pot.

One week we couldn't get our hands on pot. Our source dried up. We didn't try very hard to find another. We just switched to beer temporarily, we said. I didn't much care. I figured beer would make me feel just as good, and if it didn't, I would try something else. I did, but it wasn't a new drug. I got a new boyfriend, Todd.

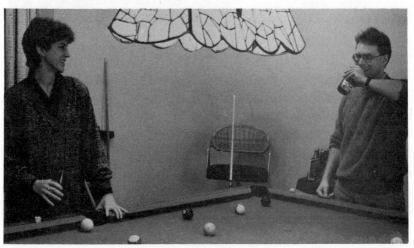

I was in love. Todd was part of the trendy, very "in" Cambridge college crowd. He had a beautiful red sports car, played saxophone in a rock band on Friday nights and could talk anybody into anything. A funny guy, right out of a television situation comedy. We did a lot of drinking together. We slept together. I was fifteen, but I was living the life of a college senior and loving it. I didn't give my classmates a thought. I rarely had my senses clear enough for thinking.

One night as Todd and I were about to begin one of our weekend binges at his fraternity house, I asked myself: Why am I doing this? My answer: I have to do this. I knew it wasn't a good thing. But I liked it too much to stop.

I had only been experimenting: a little beer, some pot. With alcohol especially it's a fuzzy line. You take a sip here and there and then you go out drinking with your friends and then it seems out of nowhere you're over the line. I was an addict at fifteen. It was already too late. I liked it. I really liked it. I didn't care why I liked it; I wasn't going to stop. I was smoking pot every day and drinking beer every weekend.

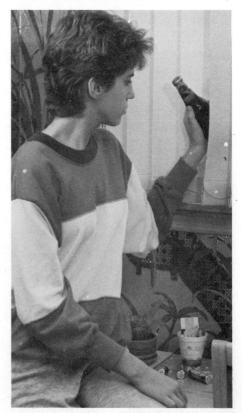

After two years of Todd's fast pace, I stopped dating him and hanging around with his slick friends. I didn't belong there anyway. Pot stopped working for me; my real self came through: I wasn't sophisticated. I was shy and very timid in spite of my imposing height and older looks. If I put on tight shorts and a tight T-shirt I could walk into any liquor store and buy all the beer I wanted. So why did I need Todd?

I found a quieter group of friends my own age, but from anoth
school. We drank afternoons, on weekends and some nights if
could sneak it. I kept emergency beer hidden behind the curtain on
my bedroom windowsill during the winter. My parents never found
the beer, but they had caught on to my drinking. They didn't know
what to do.

That frightened me. If my parents couldn't deal with this, how
was I supposed to know what to do? Handling my compulsion to
drink and smoke was the first thing in my life that they had not been
able to teach me to do. I was going to be pretty much on my own
with this one.

They became very strict and overprotective my last two years of
high school. That was probably the only thing they knew to do, I was
forced to control my drinking to some extent until I left for college.
No doubt this delayed my downfall: I was too into drinking to think
about stopping. Although pot had stopped working for me, I still
smoked it. I spent every cent I had on pot and beer.

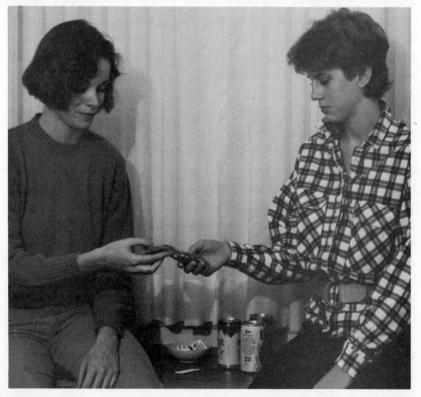

Alcohol and marijuana did the trick for me from my beginning drinking and smoking days when I was in eighth grade with Jerry. Those early years my tolerance was very low, but by college it was built way up. I drank more than ever because my parents weren't around. I could drink endlessly with friends or by myself. I would just drink on and on and on.

I knew something was wrong with me, but I didn't know what it was. I think I needed a big sister or close friend who cared about me. If someone had told me I was an alcoholic, that I had a disease, I might have stopped. I never knew what was happening.

Sometimes I would drink until I threw up or passed out. I often had to have someone stop the car because I couldn't hold my urine from all the beer. Sometimes I got incoherent, sometimes I had to be carried to my room, sometimes I threw up on people's porches and went back and drank more. I lost coats, sweaters, keys, wallets, watches, most of my jewelry. I either left them places or they were taken. I never could remember.

In the year and a half I was in college, my grades steadily dropped. I drank around the clock: days in my dorm, nights in bars until I finally went crazy or appeared to be crazy. I didn't want to drink but was going to the bars anyway. I couldn't stop myself from leaving my room.

I was broken. I was alone. My drinking friends weren't covering for me anymore. They weren't helping me get back to the dorm. They didn't even want to be with me. I lost everyone's trust. I didn't feel honest anymore.

I realized I was never going to be an important person. I was a nothing. I was in bad physical shape. My nerves were shot: I jumped when the telephone rang, when someone dropped a book, when a door shut. My body ached; my head felt as if it were going to split open most of the time.

I think mixing drugs like pot and alcohol speeds up the disease. Maybe that's what happened to me. One night I lost it: I was out of control, screaming, beating on the doors in the dorm, cursing, hitting myself. The dean took me to a hospital. The door at the end of the corridor was locked; my windows were barred. I stared at the walls and ate with the crazies. Real nuts. I screamed if one of them

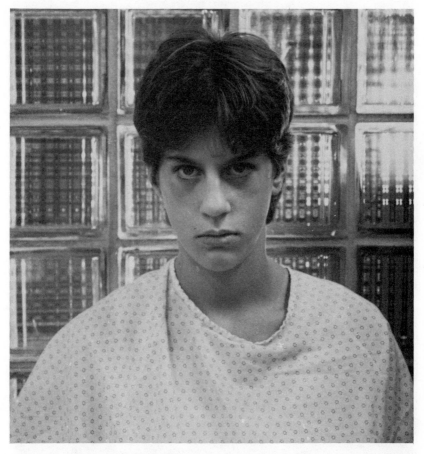

came near me or tried to talk to me. I was there three days before my parents could get me out.

My parents took me directly from the hospital to an alcohol rehabilitation center. It took a while to get me down to planet earth and to get me back to some kind of sane behavior. Once I had regained my ability to listen and understand, I was educated about alcohol. I realized I had serious problems. For the first time, probably since eighth grade, I felt a yearning to be moral.

I was willing to do what it took to stay sober. After the rehabilitation program, I joined AA. AA means commitment and time. The recommendation is ninety meetings in ninety days to get acquainted with their program. I went. I still go. I also saw a psychiatrist daily for two and a half years.

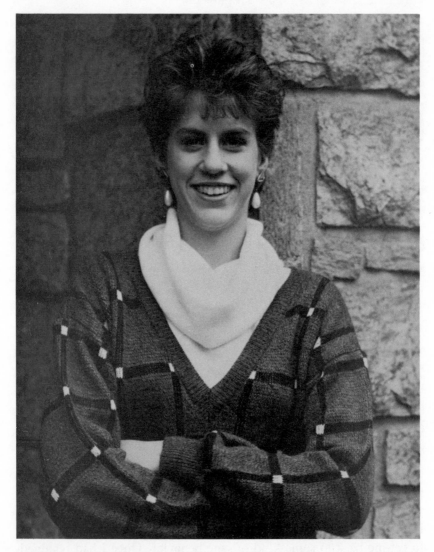

I was only drinking beer and smoking pot when I hit bottom. I thought they were harmless. If only I had known. It took me a long, long time to recover. My parents stuck by me. That helped, but I had to do the work of relearning who I am and growing up by myself.

Today my life is terrific. I have rediscovered my value system and learned that I am important, that I fit in, that I have many, many qualities and assets to offer. I have wonderful new friends, a good job and will be starting college again this fall. A clean slate in a new school.

YOU SHOULD KNOW

1. By definition, any chemical substance that changes a person's behavior or ability to function is a drug. Therefore, marijuana is a drug.

2. The impact of addiction is very troublesome whether the drug is marijuana or cocaine. If someone *needs* a joint in the morning, a shot in the afternoon or a snort at night, she is allowing a drug to control her life.

3. The drug alcohol has one known chemical. Marijuana, by contrast, has over 450 chemicals, some of which alter thinking and some of which harm different parts of the body.

4. Pot smoking has very definite side effects: a constant cough and chest pains. It is much worse for the lungs than cigarettes because pot contains more cancer-producing chemicals. And we know for a fact that cigarettes cause lung cancer as well as cancer of the mouth and throat.

5. For complex biological reasons marijuana harms male sperm and female egg-cell development. That could create serious problems for people when they are older and ready to have children.

6. In the brain marijuana causes cells to divide more slowly and to have more defects than normal. This is why potheads very often have poor memories and cannot think as fast as those who do not smoke marijuana.

7. Fifty pot smoking students between the ages of 13 and 18 who were stoned at least two or three times a week during a four-month period were studied. The results are startling:

  · Their brain wave movements were immature for the students' ages and showed signs of impairment.

· When they were challenged, none of the students could speed up to do an academic task. Their brain waves did not react in the expected, normal ways.

8. Because it can take a month or more to get the chemicals from one joint out of your system, weekly or daily pot smokers collect these poisons at alarming rates.

9. Anyone who believes pot cures cancer or cleans out lungs after smoking cigarettes is wrong. These are myths. Pot does none of these things. The chemical compound THC, which is found in marijuana, has been used, but in a very pure state and in man-made pill form, to reduce the nausea that often accompanies cancer treatments, but it is not a cure for this disease.

10. Smoking pot and drinking will not make anyone more popular. It only feels that way. These drugs push down and dull true feelings. Under their influence a person can believe she fits in; feelings of nervousness and insecurity disappear temporarily. As the alcohol/drug wears off, the feelings return.

THINK ABOUT

1. Although all the evidence about the damaging effects of marijuana is not in, there is enough to know that regular use causes many different kinds of problems. Not too many years ago people thought cigarette smoking was safe.

2. The marijuana that is sold today is much stronger—some say 6 to 30 times stronger—than what was sold ten years ago, and most of it is much stronger than the pot used in scientific experiments.

3. Of the thousands and thousands of scientific tests and studies on the effects of marijuana, *not one* hints that marijuana might be harmless.

4. On top of the physical damage to lungs, liver, brain and reproductive organs, pot interferes with performance in school, increases depression and causes irritability in its regular users. These things are for sure.

5. Some things can't be changed by escaping into oblivion. Alcohol and drugs may make a person feel thinner, shorter, prettier, smarter, less shy or more part of the group. Once they are sober, most people feel the way they did before, maybe worse.

6. It's much smarter to find help for a problem or an embarrassing situation than to try to bury it with drugs.

7. Stopping an addiction is extremely difficult; for some, impossible. Addiction becomes so strong that most people cannot stop by themselves. They need help from doctors, special groups and family.

8. Many people who are addicted require medical care and hospitalization because withdrawal from drugs can be dangerous and frightening. Getting sober and getting straight can—and often does—take years.

7

■

GARY

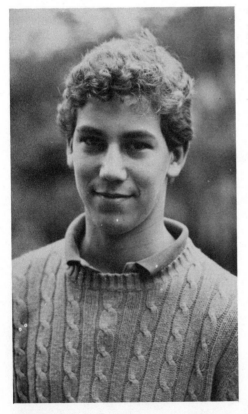

Gary's mother is a lawyer; his father, a doctor. They had an unrealistic hope he would go east to Harvard or Yale. Gary used different substances for five years and was arrested eight times before he understood he wasn't going to make it unless he stopped. According to Gary, "Before I finished, I had been on everything except roller skates."

■   ■   ■

My parents believed that if they allowed me to drink at home, I would not drink outside. I began drinking at home at age fourteen, but I didn't crave alcohol or see drinking as being grown-up. That summer we spent seven weeks at the beach and I fell in with a crowd that was drinking and smoking marijuana. These weren't your basic all-American California kids who had been my friends. They were a rougher bunch, the kind most parents don't want their kids hanging around. My parents were rarely home and didn't seem to know what we were doing.

By the time I returned home to begin tenth grade, I was drinking and I don't mean having two or three beers. I was getting drunk two or three times a week and getting high on marijuana every day. Marijuana was being pushed in every corner of the schoolyard. Alcohol was available in my house and in my friends' houses. That was our neighborhood. Our parents had booze and we just took it whenever we wanted.

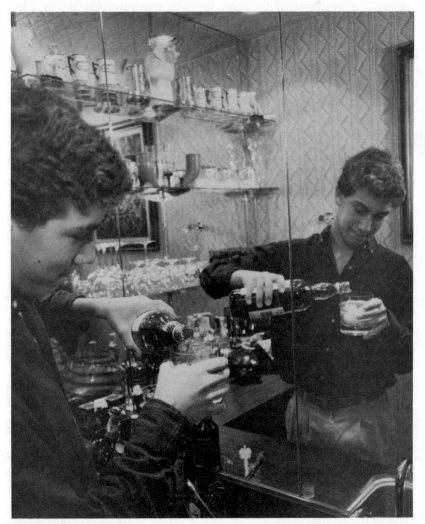

I turned on my younger brother and sister to pot and hashish. We sat in my bedroom and smoked. Whenever I had pot, and that was usually every day, I was more than willing to share with them. They looked up to me because I was older, popular, a man's man (that's what I had thought), and because I associated with people who were known to be tough and cool.

My parents, when they were home, constantly discussed my Cs, Ds and Fs. They never let up on me about my grades. My brother and sister managed to hold on with decent grades, but I was a lazy, terrible student. By the time I graduated from high school, I was taking the basics: U.S. history, English and auto mechanics. Auto mechanics for the Harvard-bound boy! I was taking that so I could steal if I had to.

As soon as I turned sixteen, I began a string of jobs to support my habit. I worked as a dishwasher, a lifeguard, an amusement park ride operator, a short-order cook. I was spending at least forty dollars a week for pot (I smoked a full ounce each week, with help from my sister and brother) plus another forty dollars in sleazy bars.

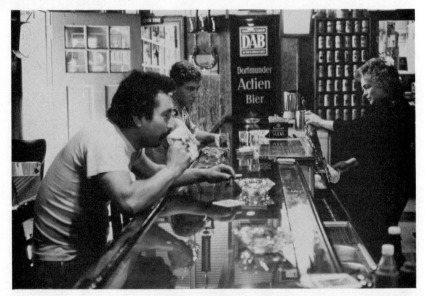

I'd go in late afternoon before the bouncer who checked IDs came on duty and drink Seven and Sevens or gin and tonics. One after another until two o'clock in the morning. I'd get smashed and hitch-hike home.

Drinking in crummy bars led to a long line of arrests for drunk and disorderly conduct and for marijuana possession. Many times the cops took me straight home instead of to police headquarters. They'd look at my library card and realize I was Dr. Hawkins's son.

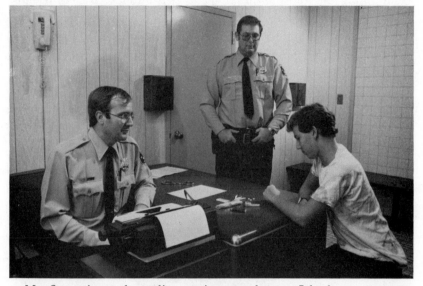

My first trip to the police station was heavy: I had to empty my pockets. They were loaded with paraphernalia: rolling papers, a roach clip, a hash pipe and a baggie with marijuana. I told my father it was the first time I had used pot. He believed me; he wanted to believe me. After that my parents were aware that I was using drugs, but since they hadn't kept a close eye on us up till then, curfews and questions stopped after a couple days.

I began experimenting with a bunch of different chemicals all at once: speed, mescaline, LSD and crack. Within a period of six months I had tried most every drug available on the street. I associated with older people who were either dealers or had access to dealers. I could get any drug I wanted whenever I wanted it.

Even though I was getting high on something before and between classes every day, I didn't think I was a junkie. After all, I wasn't sticking heroin spikes in my arm. But I began to look like a junkie. I wore tight jeans and T-shirts and kept wearing a larger and larger earring. I was a bummed-out slob who had no trouble at school because the principal was my father's patient. He was my buffer; he looked the other way.

Like school, dating was a disaster. I went out with respectable girls, the kind you bring home to mother. Girls who were straight like I used to be, never girls who were getting high. It would have been impossible to bring these "nice" girls into my circle of friends. Drugs and alcohol took priority over anyone I was dating. If someone called me up and said, "Wanna do a line of coke?" I would call my date and cancel. There was never a time—not once—that I said no to a drug.

I became a garbage mouth, especially during the summer. I would do a black beauty—that's speed—in the morning, then if a friend offered me a Quaalude—

that's a downer—I would do that at night. I'd fill in the middle of the day with gin and tonics. I didn't want to give up free drugs, although I would often black out for full days.

One night after drinking heavily in a bar I picked up a hitchhiker, beat him up and left him on the curb. I don't remember a thing about the incident other than being caught and held in jail for a few hours until the guy got cleaned up at the hospital. I was let go because he dropped charges.

By graduation I was into hash oils, which cost $250 for a small vial that lasted two days. I had to steal and deal myself to keep my drug and alcohol debts down. I had drunk away every friend I ever had. They didn't want to drink and drug the way I did. I never spent time with them and I didn't want to share the drugs I had. I preferred to keep one hundred percent for myself. People got tired of that quick.

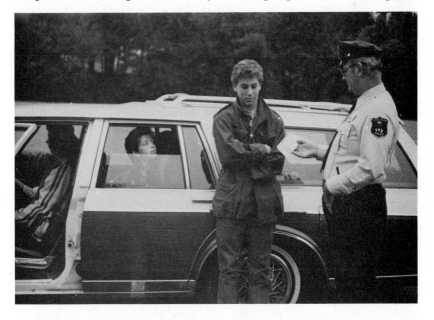

I had destroyed two sports cars in eight months and had accumulated tons of points on my driver's license. My father bought me a station wagon, thinking it would settle me. One weekend I loaded it with kids, including my sister and brother. We had two open six-packs, a quarter-pound of marijuana, a lit joint and a pint of rum in the car when I was pulled over by the state police. This cop had never heard of my father or mother.

When you're an addict, you know laws. I didn't want to do time. While he was looking over my license, the other kids in the car got rid of whatever they could. My sister was terrified; she listened to every word the officer uttered. I was booked for possession. They also should have booked me for influencing minors. I was released and went straight to a bar.

My mother went to the station house and had my charge sheet pulled and ripped up, but both parents clamped down. They started paying attention to what was going on and realized from the traffic through the house that I must be dealing. They told me I had to stop dealing or move out of the house. They were embarrassed by my clothes and attitude. They felt their reputations were being affected by my behavior. My mother told me she would not bail me out again.

They stopped working late at their offices and having dinner meetings with associates and began insisting that we have family dinners. I had to sober up to talk at dinner. It was awful; I had nothing to say. I squirmed, picked at my food and raced out of the house the instant we were excused to hit the bars. One after another.

The day I banged the side of the station wagon happened to be a day my mother came home early from court. I didn't have time to dream up a lie and at this point I probably didn't have another lie in me. I was having trouble piecing together what happened with any of my life because of my blackouts. I told her, "I think I have an alcohol problem"; not that I really believed it.

I was taken that night to an Alcoholics Anonymous meeting by a close friend of my mother's. I liked it even though I didn't do anything the members advised. I decided I could stay sober by myself without meetings. Instead I attempted a trip south to the border with a guy and stayed straight the whole way down. I lasted half a day in a motel room before diving into my friend's marijuana.

I hit the bars and joined another guy who had ounces and ounces of cocaine. A cop spotted us in the parking lot. We had white powder all over our faces and clothes. We were charged. I spent the night in jail, paid my bond and was released until my trial. I wasn't the one with the fortune in cocaine. That guy's probably still locked up somewhere.

I went home, but I knew that when I came back I might have to do

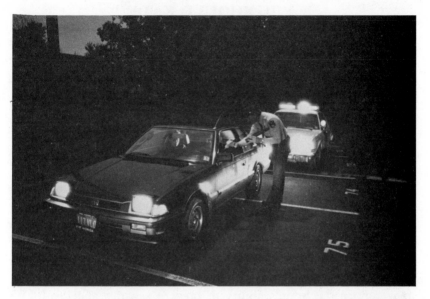

time or at the least be sent to a work farm. The judge was going to look at my record (it turns out my mother never had it pulled; she just said she did) and say, "Well, he's not a career criminal yet, but let's give this preppy boy (that's what I looked like in spite of my earring and the fact that I couldn't get into any college in the country) a taste of what it's like to be institutionalized."

I had only one option: to enter a program for rehabilitation. During my first hour the psychiatrist diagnosed me as "grossly socially immature." In those nine weeks I learned what that meant, how little I had grown in the last few years, how much catching up I had to do. I had to relearn how to eat three square meals a day, to make a bed, to care about other people.

I always feel guilty about turning my brother and sister on to pot. I thought I was being a nice guy. They could have ended up the same way I did. Fortunately they didn't.

YOU SHOULD KNOW

1. We don't know exactly why some people get addicted and others don't. Some feel that addiction is part or completely body chemistry. Others say it's part psychological makeup, part social (friends and family) situation and part or all, as pointed out earlier, heredity. Until more research is done, we can assume that for any one of us, drug dependency can be caused by one or a combination of these things.

2. With certain drugs dependency develops quickly. Crack, for example, a smokable and potent form of cocaine, hooks its users in a few months. Some crack users report being addicted after only a few "drags."

3. A recent study of animals indicates that repeated doses of cocaine may reduce the brain's ability to prevent seizures and death. We know for a fact that even a single use of cocaine can kill a person.

4. Many parents, like Gary's, help make it possible for their children to continue to use drugs. This is called enabling. Parents who pay no attention to their kids and parents who think they are protecting their children by getting them out of trouble are increasing the likelihood of more drug use and more police encounters.

5. Stealing and dealing to support a drug habit can lead to a jail term or time spent in a juvenile detention center.

6. Today kids under 18 are arrested three times more often than ever before for behavior related to their drinking and drug use.

7. Courts and schools as well as parents can commit offenders to rehabilitation programs. In Gary's case a center was his only alternative to jail.

8. Although programs vary in length from twenty-eight days to six months, most are highly structured and supervised. Some centers have comfortable living quarters; others are simple, supplying only basics. In most, patients are watched twenty-four hours a day and

rarely go home at any point during their stay. Students receive regular assignments from the schools in which they are enrolled, and tutors are provided to see that education continues.

9. Most centers conduct a series of psychological tests at the time of a patient's arrival, then place patients in appropriate groups for the remainder of their stay. Group discussions of feelings, problems, family life, events, tragedies, goals and ways to improve one's life are the focus of rehabilitation. As patients work through a program, privileges are added, but on the whole, privileges are few.

Parents and siblings are brought in for family counseling in an effort to solve problems and make changes in living patterns that may have been part of the reason for a patient's addiction.

10. Rehabilitation programs introduce patients to Alcoholics or Narcotics Anonymous, so they will have a support group once they leave the center.

THINK ABOUT

1. Drinking at home is no safer or healthier than sneaking alcohol or drugs elsewhere. Teenagers who do not drink, smoke or use other drugs *almost never* become adult abusers.

2. Each time he was let go by the police, Gary probably said to himself, "This is a breeze." He had to be faced with a jail sentence before he stopped.

3. Parents are easily fooled. They don't want to know that their child is a drug addict. Too many of them can't face such a fact or will not admit it when they do realize the truth. The easiest thing for them to do is look the other way and try to pretend that nothing has changed.

4. Gary's mother, the police and, of course, Gary felt that he was too young to be punished for what he had done. Was he? Had he been jailed or sent to a juvenile detention center for a short time, perhaps he would have reconsidered how he was living his life before it became so worthless and painful.

8

■

MELISSA

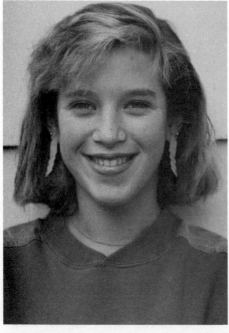

Melissa is perky and well meaning. She wants people to like her; she wants to be happy and have fun. Melissa learned the hard way that it's safer and easier to be herself. She lives with her family in St. Louis, Missouri, just on the city line, although she spent several years on her own. With help, Melissa managed to stay alive.

■　　■　　■

Somebody told me once that if you start smoking cigarettes, you're going to start doing everything else, too. It was true for me, anyway. I had my first cigarette when I was nine. I also remember thinking that if I had a beer I could never get to LSD. Now I know it's not impossible; in fact, it's real easy.

In sixth grade I switched from Catholic school to public school. There were two groups of girls in my class: the goody-goodies and the not-so-goods. Both wanted me. I loved the attention. I couldn't decide and had no one to ask. I chose the group that drank and smoked. Allison became my very best friend. We didn't do anything very exciting; we just hung out.

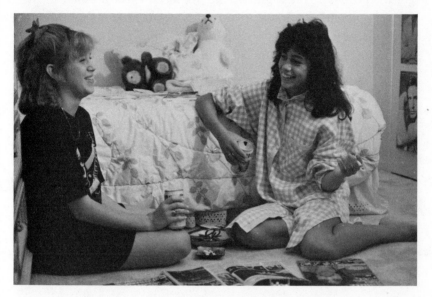

I never really liked the taste of beer, but I drank it anyway because I liked the way it made me feel. In sixth grade my tops was six beers. One six-pack made me pretty drunk. Most of the time we drank and smoked pot and got pretty wasted every weekend at Allison's house. Her parents were very liberal; she could do anything she wanted as long as she was home. I knew if I went home smelling like a cigarette and a can of beer my parents would kill me. I hated them anyway so I spent most weekends at Allison's.

There's no love in my family. For no reason, if my older brother says something my father doesn't like, my father goes over, punches him and beats him up. My dad's probably an alcoholic but doesn't know it. I can't remember the last time I told my parents I loved them or they told me they loved me except when I was in the hospital.

During the summer a new family bought the house down the street. One daughter was my age and we got real friendly. I liked Kelly because she was down to earth; she was the way I wanted to be. I liked the attention she got from boys. I loved boys, but I couldn't figure out why they didn't go after me. I always had to chase them. I followed Kelly for two years and tried to do whatever she did.

Kelly drank gin and tonics. I hated them. I had to hold my nose to get them down. One night we did six in a row at her house. Most Saturday nights we drank, then went over to Frankie's, one of the guys on our block. We stayed there until two, three in the morning and went back to Kelly's to sleep. Her parents didn't pay too much attention to where we went or what time we got home.

I had gotten used to the disgusting taste of beer and had added gin and tonics, bloody marys and screwdrivers to my menu. I only drank periodically, you know, on weekends, and occasionally whenever I felt like it during the week, usually when I was bored. I smoked pot every day.

If we weren't sitting around drinking, we were at these crazy wild parties. There was lots of pot smoking. I really loved pot and started dealing it in eighth grade. Dealing was easy. Guys just come up to you at parties and ask if you want to buy. I'd smoke half, sell half. I never made any money, just enough to buy more.

I baby-sat two afternoons a week and Saturday nights for Mrs.

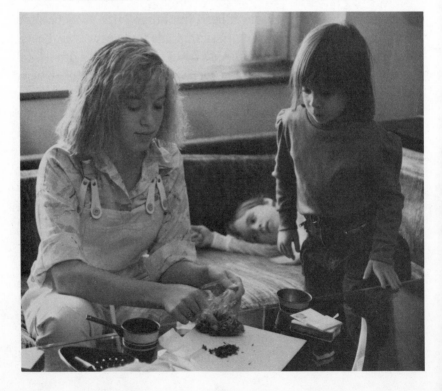

Paulson's twins to earn extra pot money. Baby-sitting was also freedom from my mother. I rolled joints in front of the twins and told them they were cigarettes. Often I invited Kelly and Frankie and a few of the older guys to keep me company. They would arrive with a case of beer and a bottle of vodka or gin as soon as I made the all-clear call.

One Saturday night we had Mrs. Paulson's house torn apart. We were crazy drunk, the music was blaring and in she walked at eleven-thirty instead of her usual one-thirty or two o'clock. My friends flew out the back door with what was left of the booze; the twins, who were watching from the stairs, flew back to bed.

The next day I apologized and told Mrs. Paulson that it would never happen again. She believed me because she had never caught me before. We continued to party at the Paulsons' until one night when I had four guys and two girls partying with me. We were stoned out of our minds, dancing and singing. The twins were watching from the steps. Mrs. Paulson took one look and never called me again.

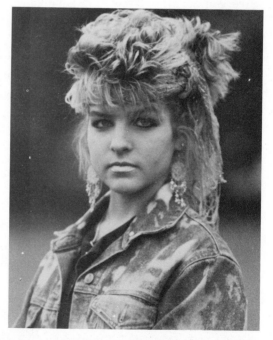

When I turned sixteen I got an after-school and weekend job. That's where I met Tiffany. We worked on the same floor in one of those big chain department stores. Tiffany was a rowdy person who, like Kelly, got a lot of attention from the guys I wanted to be with. She had a mind of her own. I liked the way she dressed and the way she acted. I didn't have enough money to dress like Tiffany or to keep up with her drinking and drugging, so I stole. For almost nine months I took cash from the register, clothes from the rack.

The store built a platform on the ceiling right behind my register for cameras. I knew exactly what was going on. I knew that I was stealing too much. I also knew I had to stop or I would get caught.

This very pleasant-looking woman handed me a twenty-dollar bill to pay for a belt. I slipped the twenty into my pocket on the way to the register to get a bag and her change. Ten minutes later a security guard and the lady came back and asked me what I had put in my pocket. A receipt, I answered. They took me, each holding an arm tightly, to a series of small, dark offices walled off from the main parts of the store.

This was the big time. They asked me over and over: "How much have you taken?" "How long have you been stealing?" I answered over and over: "I don't know." That's the answer I used with my mother, but it wasn't working with these people. They had months and months of register tapes and they knew to the penny how much I had taken, plus they had pictures of me doing it. I stuck to "I don't know" until they sent in this bruiser. He was big and he was a bully. I admitted to three thousand dollars and agreed to pay it back. He told me a police report would have to be filed and I would probably be sent to a juvenile home. I cried so hard they called my mother instead of the police.

I didn't know what to do. Nobody was going to like me anymore. I thought about running away, but I didn't know where to go. My mother was furious; she couldn't understand. "Why did you do it?" I stuck with my usual: "I don't know." It worked again. She took my savings account money to repay the store, and the incident was forgotten.

I got another job, I stole, I got fired. Job after job like that. I lied, I cheated, I stole, but I had money to buy the alcohol and drugs I needed. At one of my after-school jobs, Nick, a stock boy in my section, introduced me to cocaine. He taught me how to arrange the powder in a skinny row and sniff it up my nose. Forget it! I did that

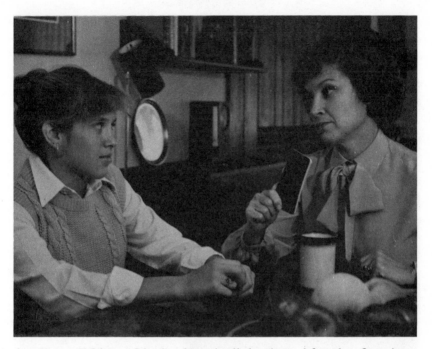

first line and I knew I had to have it all the time. After that first time, it seemed it was never ever enough.

At another job I made a new friend, Nina. She had a good head on her shoulders, and since I didn't know what I was doing and had no direction, I did what Nina did—party. Nina's friends were really scummy, but they had speed. I graduated from high school by the skin of my teeth.

After graduation I used speed and coke, drank and worked in a fast-food joint when I managed to get there. At eleven-thirty every night I dragged myself home because my father said he would throw me out if I wasn't in on time. I was a walking zombie. I didn't like myself, but that wasn't new. I had hated myself for as long as I can remember.

My parents were fighting with me because I was coming home later and later. They took my car away. I stole it to pick up some speed. When I drove up, my father was standing in the driveway. The backseat looked as if a large New Year's Eve party had just ended: open bottles of vodka, squashed beer cans and empties of all varieties on the floor. My father started yelling. I ran. I shouted disgusting things and told him I hated him.

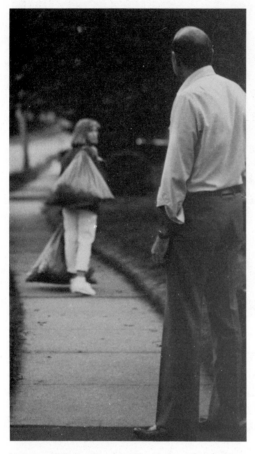

When he caught me he dragged me into the house and threw me in my room. After a few minutes my mom came in to find out what was wrong. I said, "Nothing," but this time I knew something was wrong. I wanted to tell her that I needed help. She asked me if I was having a problem with drugs. I came very close to saying yes, but I said no. My father, who had been screaming through the house about what a no-good I was, threw a bunch of big plastic garbage bags at me and told me to pack.

I dragged my stuff to a friend's place and eventually moved into a rooming house. Nobody cared and nobody wanted to take care of me. I couldn't take care of myself. I was caught up in everything else around me except my responsibilities.

My next job was back on a cash register. I stole, but they liked me enough to put me in the back of the store on a conveyor belt. As each product zipped by, I stuck a price ticket on it. I was real fast on the belt because of the speed. I liked it. I thought I was smart; I thought I knew what I was doing. I used speed and coke to get me going; I took Valium and Quaaludes to bring me down at night so that I could get up and start over again.

I was there for six months before I freaked out on the belt. I started crying and screaming, "I can't handle this crap anymore." I didn't care. I was just another burn-out. I hated myself; I wanted to die. Nobody loved me. After that I decided I had only one life to live and I might as well live it up. I convinced myself that being high was safe because you can do and be anything you want. You don't have to be yourself, but you have to have a strong head. You can get terrified by what a drug does to you—like going nuts on the conveyor belt—but when you're as far gone as I was, nothing stops you.

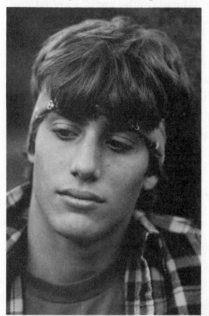

I got toasted every night, but I stayed away from guys who shot needles until George. George was a real addict who dealt drugs. With him, I could get speed or coke whenever I wanted. He did needles—spikes, they're called—but I stuck to speed, coke and alcohol. He was a sick pup. I felt sorry for him. I wanted someone to care about and wanted someone to care about me. I tried to help him and he tried to build me up, but he was a maniac.

One night on the way to where I was staying, we had a huge fight. I must have gotten on peo-

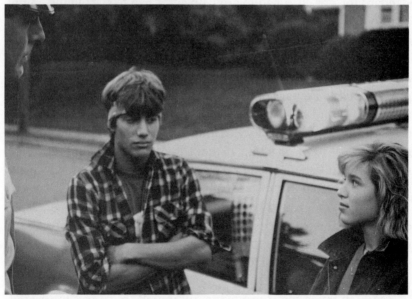

ple's nerves when I drank because whenever there was alcohol in my system I'd find myself in some kind of physical fight. In the middle of the road, George turned the ignition key off and started beating me. I have to admit, I may have hit him first. I got out of the car, and he chased me and started banging my head on the curb. I yelled and yelled and someone called the cops. I told the cop I was fine. I wanted to get rid of him before he realized we were both drunk and drugged. I was barely eighteen and didn't want to go to jail.

George's family got wise to him and sent him to a rehabilitation center. I told myself that I wasn't that bad; I didn't need rehab. I had no one. I didn't feel good enough to see any of my friends and I had lost another job. My next one was in a deli. I asked the owner's son if he did coke. We were buddies instantly. That's how I thought you made friends: if you did drugs, you were cool. I hated this guy, he was a real jerk, but I hung around with him anyway.

If I felt I was slowing down on the job, I found a little speed for energy, but I wasn't enjoying the high anymore. It was necessary. When my brain was getting fried from speed, I would drink instead. I always had something. There were times when I couldn't talk to anybody. I would run to a bar to bring me down so I could relax. I had no straight thinking, but I knew I had to set some kind of standard for myself. I had to grow up and I had to start living on my own, but I couldn't. I had to ask people for every kind of little thing because I had no idea what was right and what was wrong anymore.

Whenever I tried to get straight, I got bored and became very shy. I didn't like myself that way, but my new boyfriend did. I would promise Teddy I'd have only one beer, but after one I couldn't stop. I gave up beer and went to bloody marys, rum and Coke, or vodka and orange juice. Once while I was dating Ted, I stopped drinking for six months. Instead of drinking I smoked pot and snuck speed. I told myself I wasn't an alcoholic because I had stopped drinking for six months. I smoked pot instead and snuck speed behind Ted's back.

I couldn't understand why he was dating someone like me, especially after I started getting violent. When I drank I beat him up for no reason. I would rage. It got to the point that I could not say I was sorry anymore. Sorry didn't mean a thing, I had said it so many times.

Teddy dumped me. I wanted to kill myself, but I was too scared.

So I drank and drank. I started going to work like a slob. I didn't know where I fit in or if I fit in. My last job while I was an addict was in the warehouse of a huge chemical plant. I was so out of it, I can't even tell you what I did there.

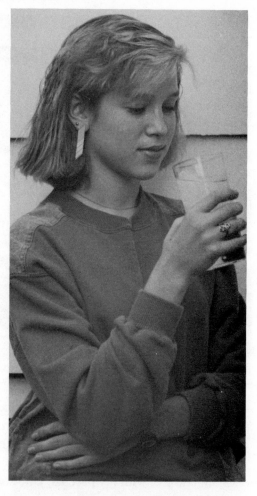

I fell asleep over some chemical crates when a co-worker tried to get me up to punch out for the day. I told her to get lost and instead of thanking her for helping me out, I punched her, swinging with all my might. I was raving. I'm sure I had Valium, speed and coke in my system at the time because I was doing them together. I ranted and moaned until someone finally called the hospital. The medics strapped me to a stretcher. I was in intensive care for three days.

I told the doctor about my drinking and drug use. She asked me if I would go into a drug rehabilitation program. I didn't think I was an alcoholic or an addict, but I had to do something. I couldn't go back home. I couldn't be on my own. I didn't know how to make it by myself . . . and didn't want to.

When I heard one of the rehab patients say she couldn't have just one drink, I admitted that was me, too. I wasn't a violent person, but when I drank I was mean, very mean—like my father. When it was my turn to speak, I stood up. Tears choked my words: "I'm Melissa. I'm an alcoholic. I'm a speed freak. I really want to die."

I went through two rehabilitation programs, during which I tried

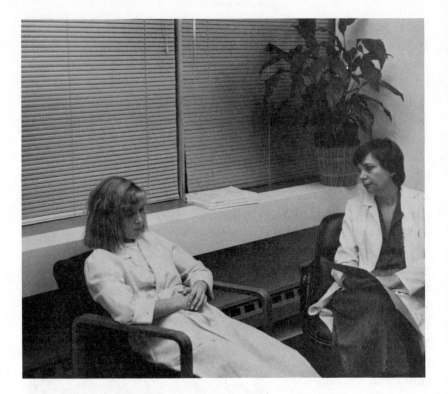

to kill myself twice. I was finally put on a hospital ward for suicidal patients. I worked with a great psychiatrist who didn't let me leave until I felt good about myself, until I liked myself.

I've been drug-free for almost a year. I work as an accountant's assistant and live with my parents, who still don't say they love me. I get furious with my father when he's drunk, but it's his life and this is mine. My parents haven't changed, but I have.

YOU SHOULD KNOW

1. The path of devastation is pretty clear-cut for most people. A person usually starts out drinking only at parties. Self-control weakens, and use is limited to parties and weekends. The boundaries widen, and one night during the week is added, then two. Finally use is daily, first at night, then starting earlier and earlier in the day.

2. When a person increases her drinking schedule, she increases the amount she drinks. What started out as an occasional can of beer or joint at a party blossoms into strong addiction.

3. There is no trick to getting your hands on drugs, but finding the money to pay for them can lead a person to a place she doesn't want to be. Older friends and parents may be the suppliers in the very beginning. As tolerance increases, the drugs received from others are not enough.

Theft often becomes the way to pay for the larger quantities required. Getting money for drugs also becomes more important to the addict than any of the consequences of stealing.

4. Drugs push pain and feelings away, making day-to-day conflicts easier to deal with for a short time. But people must *feel* both good and bad in order to grow up and learn how to handle problems. As she got older, Melissa became helpless because she had faced very few difficult situations. Melissa had used drugs to wall off feelings that would have taught her to be competent and self-assured.

5. Alcoholics have a hard time accepting the fact that they are addicted. After they admit their problem to others, they still cannot admit it to themselves.

6. Alcoholics and drug addicts like Melissa begin to think that they are losing their minds. Having a desire to kill themselves is very common. Many attempt to take their own lives. In fact, it is believed that the suicide rate is *32 times* greater for alcoholics than for other people.

THINK ABOUT

1. Melissa wanted to be someone else: first Allison, then Kelly, then Tiffany. She didn't want to be Melissa. She was influenced by others because she felt they were better than she was. The better a person likes herself, the less likely she is to hide behind drugs.

2. Not everyone can be a great soccer player or the best dancer in the class. In our own way, each of us has special qualities and talents: being very considerate of others, baking fabulous cakes or taking excellent care of a brother or grandmother. Someone could be good in science or be a whiz at writing English papers. No one does everything well.

3. In some ways drugs are like potato chips: there's always a nearby place to buy them, and once you start consuming them, it's very difficult to stop.

4. Though many young people hate the taste of alcohol, as Melissa did, or throw up or are frightened by a reaction to a drug, they continue to abuse that drug. There are probably as many bad "trips" as good ones, yet addicted drinkers and druggers keep using, only to become more deeply dependent on drugs.

5. Melissa found someone else in worse shape, someone closer to the bottom. Those kinds of people are always around. That didn't mean her addiction wasn't serious. She used George as an excuse to make herself feel better and to avoid admitting her own predicament.

6. Excessive drugging is clearly destructive. Forgetting for a moment the damage it does to your body, consider the time and emotional energy that go into figuring out where the next drug will come from. A person becomes a prisoner of "the search."

7. For many young people it takes very little drug involvement to reach the point at which they can't help themselves and their parents can't help them. At that point they need experienced, trained people to work with them.

9.
STEVE

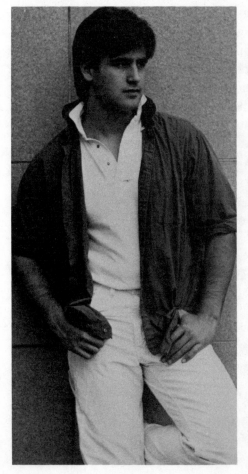

Steve has dark brown hair, dark eyes and a knockout gorgeous face. He is athletic, was a sports hero and was extremely well liked by both friends and teachers. He lives in Dallas, Texas, and comes from an affluent, well-respected, upper-middle-class family. Steve appeared to have the world at his fingertips.

■ ■ ■

I had an attitude toward drugs that my mother and school had drummed into me. In school they showed scary movies about drug users. I had a real hatred for drugs and the people who used them. I was a drinker from the beginning. I didn't think of alcohol as a drug.

My father was a strong disciplinarian and high-powered executive. We had a ton of money, lived in a beautiful house with a swimming pool, took ski vacations in Colorado and trips to exotic Caribbean islands. What people saw when we went out to dinner was the perfect, happy family: four beautiful brown-haired, brown-eyed, well-behaved children and two attractive parents. What they didn't see were the beatings my father gave us and the shouting my mother did to keep us in line. When the doors shut in our house, all hell broke loose.

On my first day in eighth grade, my father walked out; disappeared. We went from steak dinners to food stamps and from a well-kept home to one that was in total disrepair. I was angry that my father had deserted us, but no one in our family ever discussed it. We didn't talk about our feelings. I never talked about how I felt with anyone, ever. I thought it was a sin to talk about what went on behind the closed doors of your house. In a way I was relieved that he was gone because I had more freedom. I heard about kids who had grown up on the street with no parents. I felt that way too. I felt sorry for myself. I believed that because I had such a rough life, I was maturing much faster than my friends.

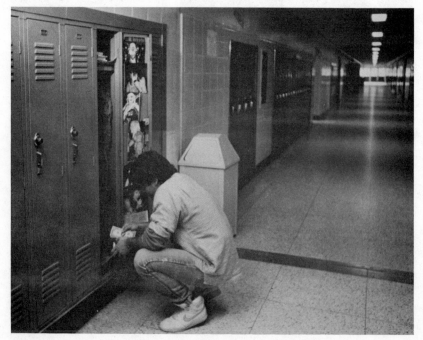

My first addiction was stealing, because there wasn't money at home anymore. I worried that there wouldn't be enough to eat. I stole wallets from the other kids' lockers. I was an excellent thief. Never got caught for that. Later I stole to support my alcohol and drug habits. I took thousands of dollars from my sisters and brothers and in whatever items were sold at the places I worked. I was arrested eight times, once in handcuffs, before I gave up drinking.

I started drinking on weekends soon after my father left. My first experience was wonderful; it was incredible. I kissed a girl. That was the good part. I embarrassed myself by urinating in the middle of her front lawn. She was looking out the window. My first kiss and my first beer made me forget the awful feeling of having been watched. I was very proud of myself.

The next few times I drank I got beat up; I threw up in a friend's basement from wine. Another time I drank fourteen beers and threw up for hours. I learned early and quickly how much I could drink to get bombed out but not get sick.

Like a street kid, I hung out with an older guy who taught me how to smoke cigarettes. He bought beer for me. In my mind, he was the greatest guy in the world. He was about twenty-seven, so I looked up to him. The age gap didn't mean a thing to me because I thought I was advanced for my age.

My brother Elliot and I drank together a lot. When he drank he attacked people and would hurt himself. He used knives. When we were together drinking, we fought. We thought brawling was part of becoming a man. Elliot and I got arrested one night for vandalizing the Christmas lights at the shopping mall. We were bombed out of our minds and climbed up on the roof. For every bulb we threw down, we put another into a shopping bag to take home for our tree. Mall security tried to stop us, but when we refused to get down, they called the police.

The juvenile officer worked with my mother, who is a drug counselor. We were reprimanded for drinking too much and sent home. Six months later I was arrested for driving a car drunk and without a license. Again I was sent home without charges being pressed because the juvenile officer knew my mother. I guess my mother knew I was going to do what I was going to do. Many nights she waited up and I stumbled in barely able to walk.

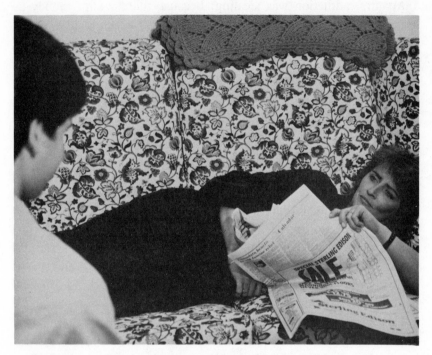

By fourteen I was already blacking out, but I could get past my mother. She made me check in. I could stand in front of her, tell her everywhere I had been, who I had been with and what we had done. The next morning I could not remember a thing I had told her.

I used the athletic field to cover up my bad feelings. Sports were my only source of self-esteem, because I was a horrible student. When I wasn't using a bad call as an excuse to fight, I was great. By tenth grade I was the rising star of the soccer, baseball and wrestling teams, but I was also drinking at odd times like Sunday afternoons on the sidelines of a football field. Considering I was a serious sports-man, it was a joke. People laughed at me, but I made sure that everyone liked me.

I hooked up with guys who were drinking like I was, but I also worked at keeping my image together as a prize jock, a non–pot smoking nice guy. My girlfriend Jeannie was very important to that image. I practically lived at her house. Her dad was home every night; they had lots of kids, and like my father, he was a tough guy. He loved me because I was an athlete. If he knew I smoked cigarettes he would have died, but he had no problem giving me beer.

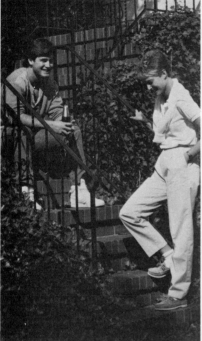

I held on to Jeannie and some of my sports glory through senior year, but after graduation my fame faded. I had the briefest stay in college—two weeks. I was picked up for stealing in the campus bookshop, taken away in handcuffs and shipped home to a job and the real world. I worked on a construction crew, drank in bars and believed that I had made it—I was a man. I still drank beer and hated people who smoked pot.

Smoking pot was the ultimate crime in my head. I saw how it had changed my friends. One of

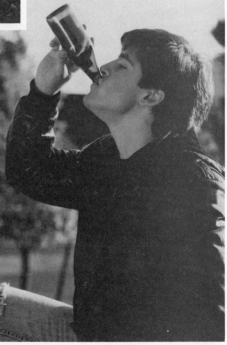

them will be in and out of mental institutions for the rest of his life. He'll never be the same. He smoked once too often. I call it getting struck by lightning. Another guy I know got struck by angel dust. He's strange and can't get his thoughts together anymore. I lost friends that way.

Finally I lost Jeannie. She and I had been together since ninth grade. When she ended our relationship, I stopped eating and playing ball with the guys on the job. I thought I had stopped living. My mother threw me out. I had no one.

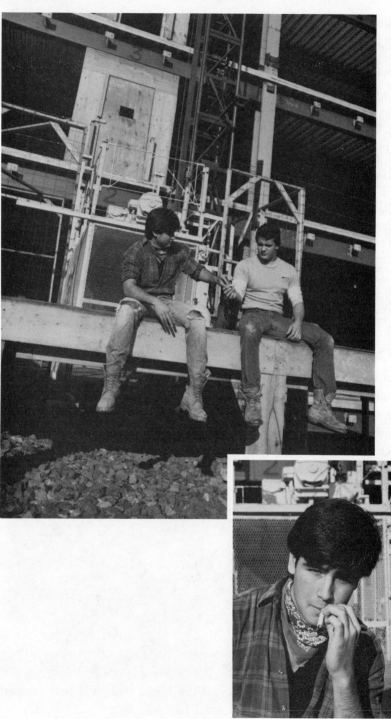

A guy at work introduced me to pot. From the first joint I became a daily user. Marijuana worked beautifully to kill the emotional pain I had about Jeannie, my mother and my father.

Pot became my best friend; I lived for it. Me, the one who was so against it, found I couldn't live without it. I adopted an I-don't-care attitude. I didn't care about my body, my job, my family, anybody. I could not stop getting high. Going to work high was dangerous because they were sending me up on beams and had me hanging out doing the tricky stuff. I liked the risk, so I never refused. Like my arrests, I got off easy with only a few trips to emergency rooms, nothing serious.

To expand my horizons I took a long trip. In Oregon I moved in with a bunch of freaky guys who were into the heavy stuff: cocaine, LSD, mushrooms and the other psychedelics. My first experience

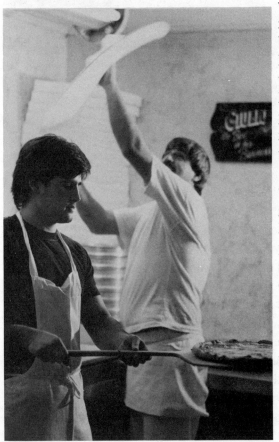

with LSD sent me into a panic. But, like beer, I learned to take less to avoid a bad trip. When I wasn't high, I was cooking pizzas and stealing money from the boss until I got fired.

I could not stomach the reality that I had gone from high school hero to out-of-work pizza pie maker. I stopped taking showers. I stopped brushing my teeth. I grew my hair long and didn't wash it. I survived by getting food stamps illegally. I knew I was in trouble; I knew I was an addict. I needed help. I went home.

I told Elliot I didn't feel well, that I had been eating LSD and that life had stopped. "Tell Mom," he said. "She'll understand better than anyone else." I told him I couldn't do that. Elliot said something I'll never forget: "Then at least stop breaking her heart." He dented my armor.

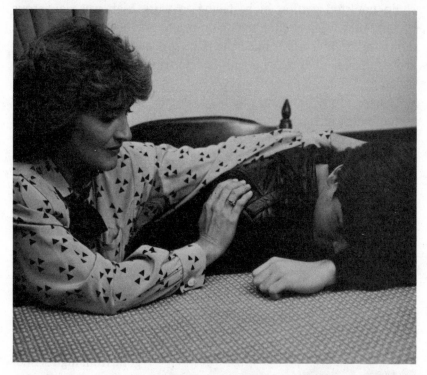

I talked to my mother. "It's coming to the end for you," she said. I couldn't accept that because I had been determined from the beginning to be a successful drinker. I wanted to drink the way I wanted to and not get in trouble. But I had a sense that I was really killing myself, that I was not going to live long.

I was suffering real physical effects. My front teeth were so loose they wiggled; my nose bled most of the time; my withdrawal shakes were like miniature earthquakes. In the morning I took cans of beer into the bathroom. I drank there because I knew I would throw up. I'd drink and throw up, drink and throw up until I got more down than up and had enough alcohol in me to get rid of the shakes. I had constant stomach pains and sore throats, but nothing stopped me.

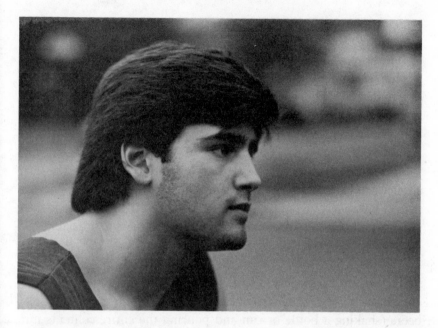

I knew what I had to do. I had to finish myself off. For the next three months I drank more in the morning; I used every drug I could get my hands on; I sold my radio, my clothes, my tapes, every possession I had. I lost my apartment, my job and finally my car. I defeated myself. I finally understood that my mother was right. I reached the end. I put myself in a rehab center.

When one of my friends found out I was there, he said, "I'm really glad you nipped it in the bud." Just shows you, no one can know what's really happening to someone else, what's really going on inside someone else's head.

Two years ago I couldn't borrow a buck to buy a beer. Two weeks ago I was put in charge of a rehabilitation program similar to the one I had entered. I'm doing something beyond my wildest dreams.

YOU SHOULD KNOW

1. The way alcohol works within the body is complicated. At first alcohol is stimulating, but its negative effects can show with only one or two drinks. Noticeable changes in behavior, such as loudness in a soft-spoken person, anger in a normally easygoing person or risk taking in a cautious person, may appear.

2. Headaches, hangovers and sleeping on bathroom floors to be near a toilet bowl are the milder symptoms of overdrinking. Add stomach pains, low energy, fatigue and sore muscles to the physical list; paranoia, depression, nervousness and sleeplessness to the emotional list.

3. Heavy drinking and chugging beers do not make you more macho. In fact, chain drinking (one right after another) and "shooting" beers (shaking a bottle or can and pouring the entire contents into your mouth at once) can kill you. What happens is the parts of the brain that control heartbeat and breathing are slowed too quickly when they receive too much alcohol too fast.

4. Blacking out is a loss of memory for a period of time. It is not the same as passing out. During early stages of blacking out, a person loses a small chunk of time—a minute, two minutes, five—in which he can appear completely normal, but later on his brain cannot tell him what he was doing during that time. The length and frequency of blackouts increase with continued drug use. Chronic abusers can black out hours, full days, sometimes weeks.

5. There comes a point when getting drugs and getting high are more important than keeping up appearances, grades, friendships, sports or physical health.

THINK ABOUT

1. Once hooked, the addict begins to get high alone just as often, in some cases more often, than with friends. His behavior or depression pushes people away because he stops being fun.

2. Some parents supply alcohol (although it is illegal to do so) because they think it is the only way they can identify with their children. They think that by drinking with the younger generation, they will be able to figure out what and how you think.

3. Even when someone believes he has buried bad feelings, he carries them and the pain that goes with them. They get stored in the back of the mind to explode at a later date. Steve, for example, was furious with his father for walking out but didn't realize it until his hurt and pain exploded during a therapy session at the rehabilitation center.

4. When someone is in a family like Steve's, he should find an outsider with whom to talk: a teacher, a guidance counselor, a drug or an alcohol support group, a friend's mother or father—someone with whom feelings and problems can be discussed. It's okay to talk about what goes on within a family, even private matters, if they are troublesome.

5. Like those of many alcoholics and addicts, Steve's problems really began when his drinking and drugging got out of control. He lost Jeannie because of his drug abuse. Jeannie's dumping him didn't really make his life any more miserable.

6. Young drinkers and druggers often think they are wiser and more worldly than other kids their own ages because they're regulars at the local bar, friendly with an older crowd. What's really happening is that they are pretending to be adults but are staying kids because the skills and feelings they need to mature are blocked by booze and drugs.

Like airplanes waiting to land, they circle, making no progress in their psychological development. When they land from their individual nightmares, they will be the same as they were before drugs.

10

■

LAUREN

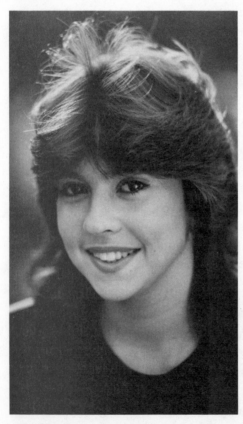

Lauren was the family baby, born in Chicago six years after her brother. Her grandparents, aunts, uncles and cousins lived in the same community. They spent weekend and mid-week time together. Lauren was cared for, loved and pampered by many people because she was the youngest.

■   ■   ■

I didn't want to leave my mother. I hung on her dress crying each morning when she took me to kindergarten. I was afraid of the kids. Once I had been pried away from her, I sat quietly, too shy to speak up or play. I didn't get these feelings again until fifth grade, when the city changed its school district lines. Most of my friends stayed in the same school, but I was switched. Many of the kids in my new school had been together since kindergarten and had formed close friendships. I was not accepted: My parents were too tall; my hair wasn't permed; my father didn't wear suits to work—who knows? They didn't like me. I hated school. I wished I were invisible so no one would know that I was there. I went through this every single day. I was terrified of people, but I forced myself to participate.

The next two years I worked hard on my piano and played a lot of soccer. By seventh grade I was so good that I was the only one my age to make the team. I was a star. Boys started to notice me, and the crowd was more accepting. But I had little time for socializing.

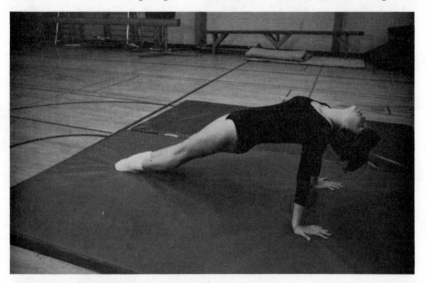

I was a competitive gymnast and practiced hours and hours on weekends. I was planning to go to the Olympics. In ninth grade my parents enrolled me in an all-girls school with an excellent gymnastics program, but I totally withdrew. I didn't try out for the soccer team; I stopped gymnastics after two months; I quit piano. I suffered through the year and returned to public school.

Cigarettes and pot were especially interesting to me because I thought they would make me acceptable to the "right" crowd. I got very high the first time before school on Halloween. The kids were passing joints in front of school. Everyone was in costume and looked strange and creepy to me. I could not find my home room or locker. That scared me so much I didn't smoke pot for months.

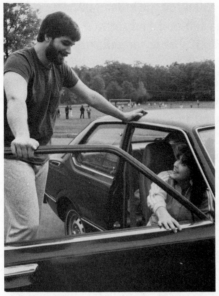

One night after soccer practice—I had started playing again—the baseball coach offered me a ride home. It took me years and years to figure out what happened that night. He was a coach, a teacher. It never occurred to me that he would do something wrong.

I didn't want to; I asked him not to; he did it anyway. I couldn't believe it had happened. My mother had never talked to me about sex. I let this guy touch me and then it got way out of hand.

After that I felt strange, cut off from everyone, different. I hated what I had done. I clung to the coach. I started drinking and drugging with him every single day. I was a fifteen-year-old who knew nothing about anything one day and the next I was thrown into black wildness: weird parties, people touching, wearing clothes, not wearing clothes, strangers, crazy-looking apartments, mirrors, nothing normal.

I was hardly ever in class. I was kicked off the soccer team for missing practice. Everything I had ever known about myself, every ideal, any concept I had about what I was like or what other people were like was gone within six weeks.

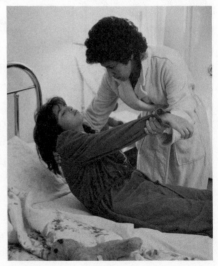

I tried to kill myself. My parents found the bottle of pills and Mother pulled me out of bed. They called the hospital to find out what to do. My mother started beating me up and shouting at me, "What will other people think if you kill yourself?" They sent me to school the next morning as if nothing had happened; to a psychiatrist the next afternoon.

After two weeks of therapy the psychiatrist said I was overanxious and prescribed tranquilizers. My parents, however, had their own methods for keeping me calm and preventing suicide. My father drove me to school, picked me up, brought me home and locked me in my room every afternoon for one solid year. Locked, with a key. They were going to show me, buckle me down.

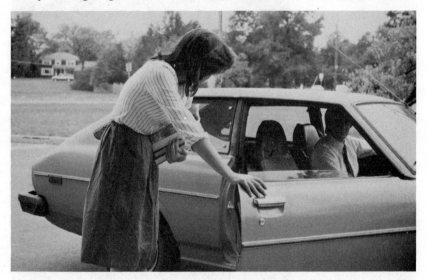

I was in so much emotional pain that I did anything I could to get away from that pain. I cut school in the middle of day, got high and was feeling pretty good by the time my dad drove up at three o'clock to jail me. Summer was easier because they couldn't keep me barred twenty-four hours a day. They kept tabs on me by putting me to work in their shoe store, but I snuck out of the house every night to get high.

If I had to sleep with a guy to get the drugs I needed, I did. I started partying with a wilder crowd. Months passed during which I thought what I was doing was cool. The more dead my brain got from dope and alcohol, the less able I was to think about what I was doing. Every now and then I woke up as I had that first time and got a good look at what was going on around me: My whole life was insane. I knew I was in big trouble and wasn't going to get out of it. Everything was closing in around me, and I wanted out.

I got out the only way I knew. I took a bunch of pills and sat in a chair waiting for "it" to happen. My ears started buzzing, real loud noises like ten thousand police sirens blasting in a small room. I was terrified. I knew almost immediately that killing myself was wrong. I tried to get to a telephone. When my mom found me she made me throw up and kept me moving when what I wanted was to sleep . . . forever.

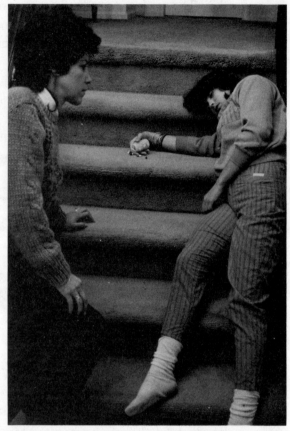

My brother, my idol, was furious and would not speak to me. My aunts, uncles, grandparents . . . everyone in the family was in a rage. They could not believe that I had the nerve to destroy our happy family. How dare I! My favorite cousin Kate, who is two years older than I am, would not stay in the same room with me. When we were together, she made a big show of getting away from me.

I promised my family that I would not end my life. I knew I was killing myself with drugs and booze the slow way, but I couldn't help that. I wanted to feel part of what was going on, but more than that, I was hooked. I was trapped in the drug bind.

When I got high, something happened to my brain cells, to my top level of thinking. I lost my ability to make choices. I operated on a lower level, the instinct level. I was mentally deficient; my thinking under drugs was that of a two-year-old. I breathed, I talked a little, but I really couldn't think.

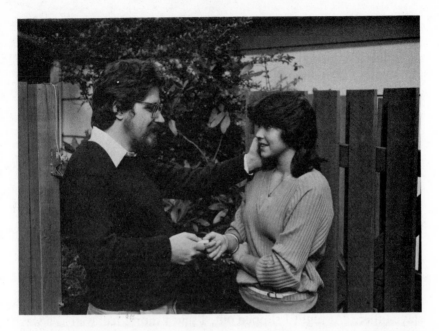

I would find a guy who had drugs and I knew only one way to get them—pot, cocaine, tranquilizers, angel dust, acid, alcohol. I did anything and everything to get my hands on drugs. My life was horrible. I always felt dirty. I always felt like a tramp. I always felt guilty. I didn't know that I could say no to men, that I was supposed to say no. Whatever the coach had told me, I did and continued to do long after he had been replaced. When I didn't like a guy, I didn't know how to get rid of him.

I spent my entire sophomore and junior years of high school on the fringes. Toward the end of summer I knew I better buckle down or I would not get into college. I stopped doing drugs and started drinking very heavily during August.

By fall I realized I was losing all my energy and decided that dragging around didn't feel very good. I went back to sports and tried to get my grades up. I needed energy so I limited myself to one glass of wine a day.

What I haven't mentioned is that every single day I was smoking pot. I had heard for so long that pot isn't a drug, that it is another tobacco. Pot doesn't harm you, it isn't the hard stuff. I didn't think of myself as a daily user, but I even smoked a couple joints the day I was put in the rehab clinic.

For almost my entire senior year I had no "hard drugs." My parents had let up on me; I appeared to be in good shape. Then one night in early spring I did cocaine at a party. It gripped me so hard. I became obsessed with it; nothing was as important as that drug. My life fell apart. I was back where I had been two years before, but it didn't matter. I wanted to stay doped up, because if I looked too carefully at my life, I would kill myself.

I wanted drugs. I was entitled, I told myself. I had worked hard. My grades were good enough to get me into college. It was time for fun. I would not admit to myself that I was addicted. I made excuses and believed them. I stayed drugged out most of the time. Sometimes I found myself in strange bathrooms, not knowing how I got there or how I would get home. After a couple of drinks, a couple of joints, I lost control and all I wanted was to find some coke.

I managed to get dressed in the morning as if I were going to school. As soon as my parents left the house, I went to my room and stayed there. At night I slipped out. I said I didn't feel well as a way to miss Sunday dinners with the family. I invented stomachaches or headaches to avoid going to church.

My mother worried about me constantly, but she could not face the truth. Twice she asked me if I was using drugs and twice I told her yes. She started swinging her arms like a lunatic and shouting, "Don't tell me that. What? Are you crazy? You are. Don't say that. You're not. I won't have it. Don't say it." After those episodes it was easier to stick to stomachache stories when she asked me how I was feeling or what was wrong. She asked a lot; I lied a lot. I was guilty and hated myself.

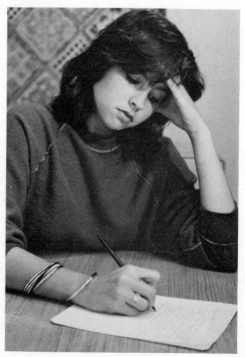

Graduation was one week away. Although I had been accepted into college, my parents were going to know very soon that I would not be part of the cap-and-gown lineup. I had not attended a single class during the last marking period. I had disgraced the family again but I couldn't face it. I started a letter to them explaining in detail what I had been doing.

My life wasn't exciting. It was the same old thing every night. Different people, a different liquid in the glass, a different thing on the mirror to suck up my nose, but it was dull. There's nothing interesting in having one thing take up your mind twenty-four hours a day, every day. Drugs and booze, drugs and booze. Selling my body. Lies. Years of lies and spending time with people I didn't like or didn't know.

Even as I wrote the letter, I was trying to scoop up the last dregs of cocaine from an empty vial. My mother was right. I was crazy. The

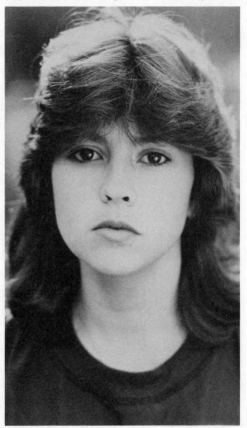

urge to kill myself returned. This time I knew I'd be successful. I called my mother at work and told her to come home immediately.

She listened and didn't listen. She still didn't want to hear. "You can't kill yourself. What will people think? Don't you move. Sit there." She told my father, who within two hours had me admitted to a drug rehabilitation clinic.

Some people look at getting straight as brave. "How courageous," they say. The truth of the matter is, if I hadn't gotten straight and I don't stay straight, I die. I have no more chances.

YOU SHOULD KNOW

1. The experiences you read—from Kim's to Lauren's—are ones you would have heard had you met any of these people in a rehabilitation center or at an Alcoholics or a Narcotics Anonymous meeting. Talking about and sharing the facts and the pain of drug abuse are a large, very important part of the recovery process.

2. It is clear from these case histories and many research studies that drinking often leads to experimenting with other, stronger drugs. Many youngsters who begin with alcohol progress to another drug or drugs and become polyaddicted. That means hooked on more than one substance.

3. Of 1100 admissions to one rehabilitation center in a two-year period, *every patient* was polyaddicted.

4. Mixing drugs is extremely dangerous. An amount of alcohol that would not get a person drunk or even a little bit tipsy by itself, when mixed with another drug (which by itself would also have a mild effect) can produce devastating reactions.

   In other words, the effects of two drugs in combination can be greater than—more than double—what might be expected. Experts believe many deaths have happened accidentally from a seemingly safe combination such as a cold pill or cough syrup and alcohol.

5. Karen Ann Quinlan, now famous for spending the last ten years of her life in a coma, became unconscious from an apparent combination of drugs. It is believed that she had popped pills, some say tranquilizers, before drinking gin and tonics. That was in 1975. In 1976 her life-support systems were turned off. However, she lived brain-dead, first in a hospital and then in a nursing home, until 1985.

6. Street drugs, those bought from dealers, are especially risky. They can look exactly like the real drug. There is no way of knowing what's been added to them that could be harmful. Many are diluted and in the process contaminated. The consequences of using such drugs can be terrible "trips" or, worse, permanent brain damage.

THINK ABOUT

1. Lauren was trapped. She didn't want to be with the coach and she didn't want to become involved with drugs. She needed to get out of her coach/drug situation right from the beginning but didn't know how.

2. When someone is under the influence, the ability to resist pressures such as sexual involvement, free drugs, dangerous dares or adventures diminishes. Defenses are down, willpower vanishes. How can someone resist if she can't hold a drink without spilling it or she's so strung out that she's afraid to leave the room?

3. Kids who drink and drug spend a great deal of time and energy lying to their parents, teachers, coaches, brothers and sisters and to themselves. The web of lies can get so tangled that the liar herself no longer recognizes fact from fiction.

4. It's true that parents can be insensitive to what's bothering their children. Some will be more concerned with what people will think than with the central problem, as Lauren's parents were. In still other kinds of families, children will drink and drug to rebel against their parents.

Whatever is going on in a particular family, no matter how parents are acting and reacting, the only fact that counts is that the drugger is hurting herself. Sure she's hurting her parents, but it's not their bodies and their minds that are getting scrambled and burned out.

5. Coming back to the world after treatment is scary and lonely. One young addict and alcoholic explained it this way: "When I got straight I had to go into a different world and interact with normal people. I didn't know how. I felt like a little girl; I still do. Lots of times I feel as if I'm play-acting. You know, pretending to be a real person."

6. Familiar friends, even family, seem strange. Feelings that may have been buried for a long, long time are exposed like fresh cuts. For the addict to escape the misery of addiction, she must often

change every single thing in her life: friends, diet, recreation, hobbies, even sleeping habits.

7. Recovered alcoholics and drug addicts have a future, but only if they stay drug free.

11

■

IF ONLY
I HAD KNOWN

Although much research and testing are being conducted, doctors have not yet been able to pinpoint who is the most likely to become addicted. They can't tell you who will cross that invisible line. There are some clues—body chemistry, heredity, psychological problems, traumatic events—but there is no surefire way to know how much drinking and drugging anyone can get away with before he has a serious problem. Some people are trapped instantly by those first drinks or drugs.

Courtney was only trying to fit in; Terry, to have a good time. Sheila was attempting to be someone she wasn't, to like herself more. Martin drank to get by in a town he hated, and Lauren got hooked in part because she lacked good information and didn't know how to stand up for herself.

Not one of them had any idea of what she or he was getting in to, how dangerous and destructive alcohol and drugs can be or how easy it is to slip back. Put another way, they didn't know hard it is to stay away from the substances that brought them down.

Kimberly hit bottom fast; Sheila, Steve, Gary, Lauren and Melissa were miserable for years. They became helpless and powerless to stop their dependency on drugs. They lost control over their lives and they lost the ability to understand and discuss their problems.

They did not know that they would change so drastically. As addicts and alcoholics, they thought, felt and acted differently. They lost their drive, their goals, their moral values and the respect of family and friends they loved and admired. It's hard work to regain all that!

There are no simple solutions to the problems of alcohol and drugs. Instead we are exposed to very powerful and very mixed-up signals. Drinking and drugging seem glamorous because television, movies, radio, books and many parents tell us to celebrate, relax, have fun or be sexy, and the way to do it is with a cocktail, a sleeping pill or a "harmless" tranquilizer.

Next time you see a beer commercial, count the ways you are being convinced that this beer is just what you need. Are the models wearing exactly the clothes you love? Are they doing things you would like to be doing? Of course, they're having the best time. Everyone is gorgeous. And yes, the product tastes delicious. And what a car! You want it.

In order to keep his or her job, the person who thought up this little advertising story is telling you that these things are possible if you drink that beer. That very same person on a different day may be dreaming up commercials to sell you insect repellent and toilet bowl cleaners.

"It's great to drink" messages make most people forget that they can refuse a drink (or drug) anytime without giving a reason or excuse. No one will argue: it's easier to accept whatever is being offered. But turning down a drink is not as hard as it used to be, because more and more of us are wise to advertising and no longer think of drinking and drugging as sophisticated. Seasoned drinkers, too, are putting the bottle back on the shelf and paying more attention to physical fitness and drug-free living.

In spite of changing attitudes among adults and teenagers, unless you have made it very clear to your friends that you don't (and will not) drink or use drugs, you will probably be laughed at, dared or challenged more than once. The better you feel about yourself, the easier it will be to resist pressure. Most of us feel our best if we have accomplished something or helped someone. Concentrate on projects and activities that you find rewarding, that provide a sense of success. Be in a play or write one. Train for and run a marathon or volunteer at the hospital after school or on weekends. Exercise regularly. Start a serious diet or a long-term project.

For the times you're bored or miserable, when the idea of taking a drink or drug could be tempting, have in mind a number of things you like to do, things that lift your spirits. They can be silly, crazy, practical or fun as long as they do the job. You may want to store one or two of these ideas in the back of your mind: see a movie, read a book, eat an ice cream sundae, take a nap, watch television, ride a bike, beat your pillow, call friends, straighten your closet, take a bubble bath or go shopping. Even a long walk, which you can take just about anywhere at any time, does wonders to clear your head and renew your energy. When you're down in the dumps, do something you know will make you feel good. But really, it's perfectly okay to feel rotten sometimes. Go off by yourself to cry or mope, or find someone who will listen to your problem.

What seems unbearable today most likely will improve. Everything changes. Someone will drop off the team you're dying to be on; your mother will get off your back; the guy or gal who hasn't noticed you yet will suddenly be the center of your life. The classes that have been so hard will become manageable. There's no way of knowing when or how something wonderful will happen. If you keep busy and move around, something is bound to happen.

On the other hand, on drugs nothing happens. One ex-addict put it this way: "When I turned twenty-one, it hit me. The last thing I remembered clearly was that I was fifteen years old. I hadn't accomplished a thing."

Drugs get in the way of goals and dreams. If you're planning to get anywhere—if you're hoping to be a surgeon or a salesperson, a stockbroker, an auto expert or a dancer—using drugs makes achieving that dream much harder, if not impossible. Another rehabilitated user warns: "If you want to blow your life away, drugs are the way to do it. Drugs rob you of everything. Take something simple like a car. If you talk about owning a Corvette or a Ferrari, forget it if you're doing drugs. You're never going to own those cars or any car."

You have learned exactly how alcohol and drugs can sneak up on you, how fast they can change your life, hurt your health, drag you down and trap you until you can't recognize yourself. Once hooked, no one gets off easily. There's no such thing as skimming the top. Almost everyone who becomes addicted, young or old, hits the very bottom sooner or later. The climb back is long, slow and tough.

In a very strong sense, you are going to be your own doctor when it comes to drugs, especially alcohol. Since no prescription is ever needed, you are responsible for your own dosage at all times. Most people respect the power of penicillin, usually taking a test to be sure they are not allergic, then taking the pills very carefully, according to directions. You have the knowledge to exercise caution around all mind-altering "medicines."

There doesn't seem to be any sound reason for dangerous levels of drinking or for using other drugs in any quantity. Look at cocaine as an example: One doctor called cocaine a loaded gun because it can stop your heart without any warning. An amount a person used with no bad effects one time could very well kill him the next time. And it has.

After refusing a few times—be it "hard" drugs, alcohol or pot—turning down drugs gets easier. Going along with the group is hardly impressive. It slots you in as just another one in the pack. You have to decide what's important to you and to do what you believe is right for you. It takes strength to be unique, to be your own person, to stand on your own and stand out.

You have just read nine cases of drug and alcohol abuse that are very serious. They are not the most tragic. None of these people turned to prostitution to support his or her habit. None is permanently hospitalized or has inflicted irreparable damage to his body. None succeeded in killing herself. Those cases are just as easy to find.

Dan is one of them. He started smoking marijuana daily in sixth grade. "I spent nine years having deep, brilliant conversations that went on and on about a rock or the color of a car or something equally ridiculous. Finally I realized that I wasn't going anywhere. Some days I shot heroin nine times. I had guys with guns threatening me because I wasn't paying my drug debts.

"I had wanted to be a doctor more than anything. I still have a lot of brain, but now I have a hard time remembering things. I have to write them down. Drugs destroyed my memory and my dream. I'll get a job, but it won't be the same. My life will never be as I had planned."

Nobody's fooling anybody. You're probably going to drink, take a few tokes on a joint or possibly sample another drug. Sometime. Somewhere. But be smart. It's very simple to believe "it won't happen to me." It's easy to ruin your life with drugs. It can be just as easy not to. Keep in mind what Courtney said: "If only I had known." You know.